本书对于中药的起源、文化、产地、采集、
贮藏、炮制、配伍、性味、归经、剂型、
剂量、用法、禁忌等进行了概述，
并将常用中药按药食同源、
用于保健食品的中药、名贵中药分为三类。

This book provides an overview of the origin, culture, producing area, collection, storage, processing, compatibility, nature and flavor, channel entry, dosage form, dosage and administration, taboos, etc., of traditional Chinese medicine, and divides the commonly used traditional Chinese medicinals into three categories: Chinese medicinals used for both medicine and food, Chinese medicinals used for healthcare food, precious Chinese medicinals.

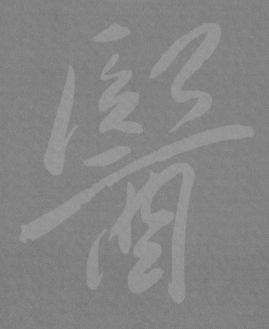

中 医
智 慧 与 健 康 丛书
TCM
Wisdom and Health
Series

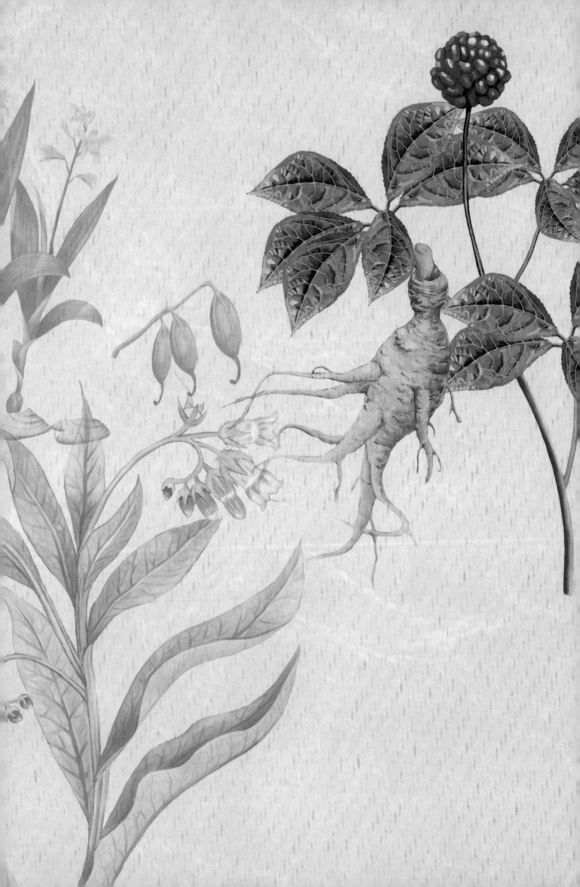

# 中华本草

（汉英对照）

# Chinese
# Materia Medica

主　编　王笑频　尹　璐　庞　博
副主编　李　奕　陈　岩　王　宜　金　敏
编　委　（按姓氏笔画排序）

王　宜　王树鹏　王桂彬　王笑频　王擎擎

尹　璐　申　倩　刘福栋　李　奕　张传龙

张曦元　陈　岩　金　敏　庞　博　姜晓晨

恩格尔　潘　雪

**Chief Editors**
Wang Xiaopin　　　Yin Lu　　　Pang Bo

**Associate Editors**
Li Yi　　　Chen Yan　　　Wang Yi　　　Jin Min

**Editorial Board**
（ Listed in order of last name stroke ）

| | | | |
|---|---|---|---|
| Wang Yi | Wang Shupeng | Wang Guibin | Wang Xiaopin |
| Wang Qingqing | Yin Lu | Shen Qian | Liu Fudong |
| Li Yi | Zhang Chuanlong | Zhang Xiyuan | Chen Yan |
| Jin Min | Pang Bo | Jiang Xiaochen | En Geer |
| Pan Xue | | | |

人民卫生出版社
PMPH　PEOPLE'S MEDICAL PUBLISHING HOUSE

**图书在版编目（CIP）数据**

中华本草：汉英对照 / 王笑频，尹璐，庞博主编
. 一北京：人民卫生出版社，2023.10
（中医智慧与健康丛书）
ISBN 978-7-117-35232-1

Ⅰ.①中…　Ⅱ.①王…②尹…③庞…　Ⅲ.①本草 –
中国 – 汉、英　Ⅳ.①R281.3

中国国家版本馆 CIP 数据核字（2023）第 189132 号

| | | |
|---|---|---|
| 人卫智网　**www.ipmph.com** | 医学教育、学术、考试、健康， | |
| | 购书智慧智能综合服务平台 | |
| 人卫官网　**www.pmph.com** | 人卫官方资讯发布平台 | |

## 中华本草（汉英对照）
### Zhonghua Bencao（Han-Ying Duizhao）

主　　编：王笑频　尹　璐　庞　博
出版发行：人民卫生出版社（中继线 010-59780011）
地　　址：北京市朝阳区潘家园南里 19 号
邮　　编：100021
E - mail：pmph @ pmph.com
购书热线：010-59787592　010-59787584　010-65264830
印　　刷：廊坊一二〇六印刷厂
经　　销：新华书店
开　　本：710×1000　1/16　印张：21.5
字　　数：421 千字
版　　次：2023 年 10 月第 1 版
印　　次：2023 年 10 月第 1 次印刷
标准书号：ISBN 978-7-117-35232-1
定　　价：158.00 元

打击盗版举报电话：**010-59787491**　E-mail：**WQ @ pmph.com**
质量问题联系电话：**010-59787234**　E-mail：**zhiliang @ pmph.com**
数字融合服务电话：**4001118166**　E-mail：**zengzhi @ pmph.com**

9

# 序

　　中医药蕴含着数千年来中华民族治病疗疾、养生保健的智慧，护佑着中华儿女生生不息，是中华民族的伟大创造与中国古代科学的瑰宝。《中医智慧与健康丛书》正是为了系统总结中医药千年来的实践经验与临床智慧、科学普及中医药知识所编撰。

　　本丛书由中国中医科学院广安门医院牵头撰写，依托国家中医药管理局国际合作司中医药国际合作专项，通过《中医史话》《中华本草》《中医诊疗》《中医养生》四个分册，全方位展示了中医药历史传承、特色优势和优秀成果，旨在向国内外读者普及中医药文化，促进中医药文化的国际传播，做好文明互鉴。丛书精心选取内容，语言通俗易懂，图文并茂，采用中英双语对照的形式，以方便国内外读者阅读。

　　我们真诚地希望通过本丛书，广大读者朋友能够更好地了解中医、用上中医、爱上中医，成为中医的"粉丝"。

《中医智慧与健康丛书》编委会
2023 年 6 月

*TCM Wisdom*

*and*

*Health Series*

# Foreword

Traditional Chinese medicine (TCM) contains the wisdom of the Chinese nation in treating diseases and maintaining health for thousands of years, and protects the endless survival of the Chinese people. It is the great creation of the Chinese nation and the treasure of ancient Chinese science. The *TCM Wisdom and Health Series* is compiled to systematically summarize the practical experience and clinical wisdom of TCM and popularize the knowledge of TCM.

This series is compiled under the leadership of Guang'anmen Hospital of China Academy of Chinese Medical Sciences (CACMS). Relying on the Special International Cooperation Project of TCM of Department of International Cooperation of National Administration of Traditional Chinese Medicine, the series shows the historical inheritance, characteristic advantages and outstanding achievements of TCM in an all-round way ranging from history, materia medica, diagnosis and treatment of TCM to health cultivation, aiming to popularize Chinese medical culture to readers at home and abroad, promote the international communication of Chinese medical culture as well as mutual learning among civilizations. The series carefully selects content, uses language easy to understand, illustrates texts with pictures, and adopts the bilingual form of both Chinese and English to facilitate readers at home and abroad.

We sincerely hope by reading this series readers can better understand TCM, use TCM, and fall in love with TCM, and become the "fans" of TCM.

Editorial Board of *TCM Wisdom and Health Series*

June 2023

# 前　言

本书对于中药的起源、文化、产地、采集、贮藏、炮制、配伍、性味、归经、剂型、剂量、用法、禁忌等进行了概述，并将常用中药按药食同源、用于保健食品的中药、名贵中药分为三类。由经验丰富的专家团队精心挑选 33 味居家常用中药进行介绍，每味中药又细分为广医药师谈选药、广医医师说功效、广医专家话食疗等话题，内容丰富，语言生动，力求兼顾实用性和有效性，便于中医药文化在海内外的传播发展。本书以汉英对照形式编写，海内外读者在系统性、全面性认识中华本草的同时，能够快速上手，走进、了解、使用简单的常见中药。阅读本书不仅能学习中华本草文化，还能掌握中药基础保健知识，以指导日常食疗与养生。

本书虽已付梓，但只是抛砖引玉。我们期待各位读者对本书的缺点和错误及时指正，您的帮助和鼓励是我们进步的动力。

《中华本草》编写委员会
2023 年 6 月

# Preface

This book provides an overview of the origin, culture, producing area, collection, storage, processing, compatibility, nature and flavor, channel entry, dosage form, dosage and administration, taboos, etc., of traditional Chinese medicine, and divides the commonly used traditional Chinese medicinals into three categories: Chinese medicinals used for both medicine and food, Chinese medicinals used for healthcare food, precious Chinese medicinals. 33 commonly used healthcare Chinese medicinals are carefully selected by an experienced team of experts. Each medicinal is subdivided into topics such as Drug Selection by the Pharmacist, Efficacy Told by the Doctor, Diet Therapy Recommended by the Doctor, etc. It is rich in content and vivid in language, and strives to give consideration to practicality and effectiveness, so as to facilitate the spread and development of traditional Chinese medicine culture both home and abroad. This book is compiled in both Chinese and English, overseas readers can quickly get started, walk into, understand and use simple common traditional Chinese medicinals while systematically and comprehensively understanding Chinese materia medica. By reading this book, readers can not only learn Chinese herbal culture, but also master the basic healthcare knowledge of traditional Chinese medicine to guide daily diet therapy and health preservation.

Although this book has been published, it is only a valuable introduction. We expect readers to correct the shortcomings and mistakes of this book in time. Your help and encouragement are the driving force for our progress.

Editorial Board of *Chinese Materia Medica*
June 2023

目录

Contents

目　录

Contents

# 目 录

Contents

# 中华本草

（汉英对照）

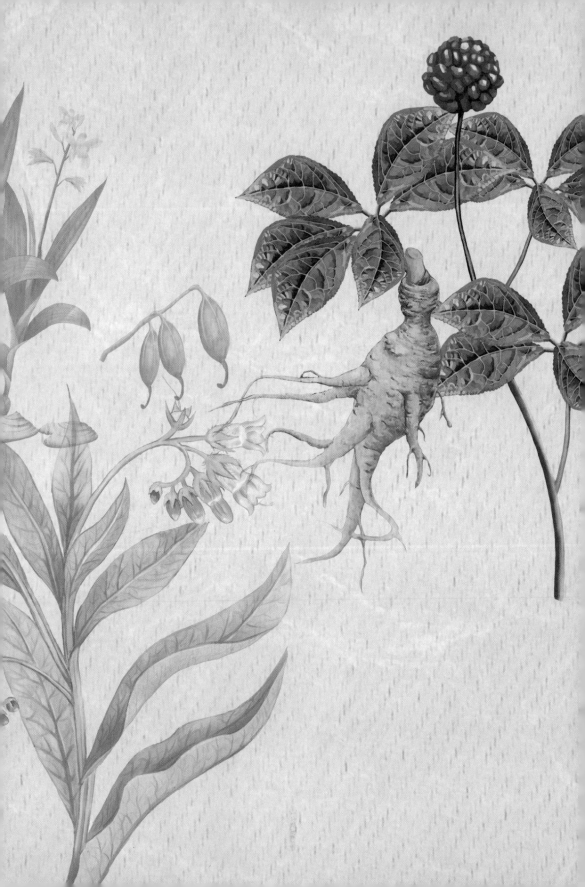

第一章

中药一般常识

# 第一节
# 中药的起源发展与文化内涵

中药历史悠久，在远古时期，我们的祖先依靠野外获取食物，常接触到各类本草，也就是我们常说的中药。其中一部分中药具有毒性甚至剧毒，但经过千百次的实践经验，这类药物的功效或毒性得以被人们口口相传下来，我们的祖先也逐步积累了区分药物与食物的经验。远古时代，人类风餐露宿，患病者十之八九，而在不经意间吃到的某些动植物可缓解相应的症状，这就是早期药物的发现过程。可以说中药的原始起源基于生活实践，而随着人类文明的日益发展，文字的创造与使用，酿酒与汤液的发明，人们在理性的思考下发现，不同的药物有着不同的功效，而不同的食用方法、炮制手段，也对中药的功效有着重要的影响。中国现存最早的本草专著当属《神农本草经》，其载药365种，依据药物的功效及对人体作用的不同，分为上、中、下三品，《神农本草经》虽作者不详，成书年代也无定论，但我们可以确定的是全书上、中、下三品的分类方法揭示了早期人们对药物的基本认识。同时在那个年代，人们已经认识到药物的四气五味、配伍方法及剂型分类，我们不禁感叹，在距今几千年前的古代中国，人们对中药的认识已经达到如此精细的程度。而后中药学又经历代发展，已经成为一门体系完备、框架完整、内涵丰富的学科。

中药文化是中国传统中医药文化的关键分支及重要组成部分，是中华文化宝贵的历史财富。中药文化不仅体现古人的医学思维，同时也蕴含着极为丰富的哲学理念，而这也是深植于中华民族文化内涵之中的核心组成部分。古人援物比类、望象取义，基于临床实践与其独有的中医思维方式，发现了药物不同的作用，如红色药入心，青色药入肝，黄色药入脾，白色药入肺，黑色药入肾，清灵的花、叶常用于治上焦病症，沉重的种子、矿石、贝壳常用于治下焦病症。正是这种独特的思维模式指导了中药的临床应用，数千年来护佑着中华民族的健康。中药是中国古代医学文化中璀璨的瑰宝，中国及世界其他国家已对众多中药开展了临床和基础研究，这些研究无不验证了中国古代医学家对中药功效的认识，并进一步推动了中药学科的繁荣发展。着眼于当代，在抗击严重急性呼吸综合征（SARS）、新型冠状病毒感染（COVID-19）的过程中，中药更是发挥了扶正祛邪的重要作用，其在干预重症转化、缩短转阴时间、提高治愈率方面均有显著作用。随着人们对健康认识的转变和养生保健需求的不断增长，中医药进入了全面发展的新时代，未来将为世界人民的健康福祉做出更多的贡献。

# 第二节
## 中药的产地、采集与贮藏

除少数人工制品（如人工牛黄、人工麝香）外，绝大多数中药都来自于天然的动物、植物或者矿物，中药或深藏于林间，或习见于田野，或隐藏于岩穴，或见于深海。因各类中药生长环境不同，且不同的生长环境会极大地影响药物的功效，因此我们将产地优越、质量优良的中药材称为道地药材，这来源于中药生产和中医医师的临床实践，并历经数千年来被无数的中医临床实践所证实，是源自古代辨别中药材好坏的一项标准。道地药材往往药效较好，现代研究也证实道地药材的有效成分要明显高于同类中药。

不同的中药都有其独特的采摘季节和储存方法，按照药物种类、用药部分可分为以下几类：

**全草**：全草类中药的采摘往往在植物生长发育最为旺盛的季节，如春夏之季。药用含根者，采摘时应连根拔起全株中药，同时要注意保护好根须，不可用力过度，以免造成对植株的损伤，影响中药功效的发挥。全草类中药储存要注意把握好温度与湿度，同时储存空间要大，以免造成对中药的过度挤压，损伤全草。

**花、花粉、叶、根**：花类及叶类药物也应注意采摘的季节，如花类药物采收时要注意采摘还未开放的花蕾或刚刚开放的花朵，此时中药的效果最佳；花粉类中药采摘，要在花朵盛开时摘取，此时能够采得的药物最多；采摘叶用中药时，要注意在植物枝叶茂盛的时候采摘，此期叶子中含有的有效成分最多；根类中药的采摘要注意采摘的手法轻柔，不要损伤根须。花、叶、根类中药的储存尤应注意对湿度的把握，以免造成中药的发霉、变质。

**树皮、根皮**：树皮类药物的采摘最适宜的季节为夏季，此季节植物生长旺盛，全株植物浆液含量充足，含有的有效成分也较多，采摘树皮也能在最低程度上减轻对植物的损伤；对于根皮，采摘季节应为秋季，此期根部生长状态最佳。储存时应注意避免虫蛀。

**动物药**：大部分的虫类药物如土鳖虫、斑蝥、全蝎、地龙、蝼蛄等，捕捉季节应在夏末秋初，此期气温较高，环境湿度较大，宜于虫类的生长，是捕获的最好季节；桑螵蛸为螳螂的卵鞘，露蜂房为黄蜂的蜂巢，此类药物多在秋季卵鞘、蜂巢形成后采集；部分动物药如蛇蜕为乌梢蛇等多种蛇类蜕下的皮膜，因对其无损伤性，故只要蛇类蜕皮时就可以采收。虫类药阴干时多质地脆弱，储存时应注意避免积压损伤。

**矿物药：**成分较为稳定，全年皆可收取，不拘于时。在阴凉、通风处储存即可。

# 第三节
## 中药的炮制

传统中药炮制的方法包括修治（纯净药材、粉碎药材、切制药材），水制（漂洗、浸泡、闷润、喷洒、水飞），火制（炒、炙、煅、煨），水火共制（煮法、蒸法、炖法、淬法），其他制法（制霜、发酵、发芽、精制、药拌）。中药炮制的目的可基本概括为减毒增效，如利用甘草水煮草乌、川乌，醋煮甘遂等可起到减毒效果，而大黄酒制、麻黄蜜制等可起到增效效果。

此外、炮制的过程也是分拣纯净药材，区分药物等级的过程，无论是泥沙类较多的中药还是冬虫夏草、鹿茸等需要依据品级定价的贵重药材，对药物的分拣都是中药上市前的重要工作。而在药物处理方面，干燥、切片、矫味都是中药炮制的关键环节。

# 第四节
## 中药的配伍

中医治病最大的特点就是把多种中药互相配伍，最终构成我们所熟悉的由许多味药物组成的汤药。北京协和医院已故名医祝谌予先生常说"用药如用兵"，如果把每味药看作一个士兵的话，那么兵种之间如何搭配、比例如何把握等成了用兵的学问，而用药也面临同样的问题。

在成百上千种的中药里，如何去了解不同药物相配疗效是提高了，还是降低了？毒性是降低了，还是增加了？我们的古人在数千年的医疗实践中，对不同药物配合应用可能引起的结果进行了长期观察，把单味药的应用与药物之间的配伍关系总结为七个方面，称为药物的"七情"，早在中国现存最早的中药学专著《神农本草经》中就有记载。"七情"包括单行、相须、相使、相畏、相杀、相恶、相反，除单行外，均生动形象地描述了两种药物配伍的关系，而中医看病处方，药物配伍应用的原则也多从这里得来。

所谓**单行**就是指用单味药治病，适合于病情比较单纯的情况，所以可以选用一种针对性强的药物，如单用一味黄芩治轻度的肺热咳嗽等。

**相须**是指性能功效相类似的药物配合应用，可以增强其原有疗效。比如有时候许多便秘患者即便吃了大黄也没有效果，但是加上一种神奇的药粉——元明粉，就能达到立竿见影的效果。

**相使**是指性能功效方面有某种共性的药物配合应用，以一种药物为主，另一种药物为辅，以提高主药疗效。如清热泻火的黄芩与通腑泄热的大黄配合时，大黄能提高黄芩清热泻火的疗效。

**相畏、相杀**则是指通过配伍可以减少其中一味药的毒副作用。比如生半夏和生南星的毒性能被生姜减轻和消除，所以说生半夏和生南星畏生姜，也可以说生姜杀生半夏和生南星的毒。

**相恶**是指两种药物合用，一种药物与另一药物发生作用而致原有功效降低，甚至丧失药效。如人参恶莱菔子，一般认为莱菔子能削弱人参的补气作用。

**相反**则是指两种药物合用，能产生毒性反应或副作用。如中药中所说的"十八反""十九畏"中的若干药物配伍就是。

中药"七情"之中，不合理配伍实际上只有相恶、相反两种。临床上应用中药复方汤剂治病时，尤其是我们在居家食疗的过程中，更要注意学会搭配，不仅要让药物适合自己的体质和病证，更要学会食材、药材之间的合理搭配，达到增效减毒的效果。

# 第五节
## 中药的用药禁忌

中药虽相对安全有效，但在日常生活及临床用药的过程中也应注意中药的用药禁忌，其主要包括配伍禁忌、证候选药禁忌、饮食禁忌、妊娠禁忌等。

配伍禁忌主要为中医学用药认识到的"十八反"和"十九畏"。"十八反歌诀"最早见于金代张子和《儒门事亲》："本草明言十八反，半蒌贝蔹及攻乌，藻戟遂芫俱战草，诸参辛芍叛藜芦。""十八反"是指乌头（包括草乌、川乌、附子）反半夏、瓜蒌类中药（瓜蒌、瓜蒌皮、瓜蒌子、天花粉）、贝母类中药（如浙贝母、川贝母、平贝母等）、白蔹、白及；甘草反海藻、大戟、芫花、甘遂；藜芦反参类中药（如人参、党参、西洋参、丹参、玄参、苦参、南沙参、北沙参等）、细辛、白芍、赤芍。"十九畏歌诀"最早见于明代刘纯《医经小学》："硫黄原是火中精，朴硝一见便相争，水银莫与砒霜见，狼毒最怕密陀僧，巴豆性烈最为上，偏与牵牛不顺情，丁香莫与郁金见，牙硝难合京三棱，川乌、草乌不顺犀，人参最怕五灵脂，官桂善能调冷气，若逢石脂便相欺，大凡修合看顺逆，炮燀炙煿莫相依。""十九畏"具体指：硫黄畏芒硝，水银畏砒霜，狼毒畏密陀僧，巴豆畏牵牛，丁香畏郁金，芒硝畏三棱，川乌、草乌畏犀角，人参畏五灵脂，肉桂畏赤石脂。

证候选药禁忌主要因为药物具有偏性，从阴阳角度看，有寒性药、有热性药，从升降角度看，有偏上升的、有偏沉降的，从补泻角度看，有偏补、有偏泻的。中药应用的核心在于纠正人体的偏性，若临床诊疗不当，应用失误，即药不对症，则可能会加重病情。

所谓饮食禁忌，即在服用中药的过程中应采取的对某些食物的禁忌，如常规忌食生冷、油腻、刺激性食物。中医学认为，生冷食物会抑制人体阳气的生发、困遏胃阳，油腻食物容易生痰，造成病理产物的蓄积，刺激性食物易耗气动血，此三类食物都会在一定程度上影响疾病的康复过程，延长患病时间。

妊娠用药禁忌是指部分中药具有损害胎元、诱发小产的副作用，因此对于孕妇，凡是对母体不利、对胎儿不利、对产程不利者皆禁止应用。其包括含有毒性的中药（如牵牛子、雄黄、川乌、马钱子、猪牙皂等），活血化瘀、行气之力较强，或具有滑利之性的中药（如桃仁、红花、大黄、肉桂、瞿麦等）。

# 第六节
# 中药的剂量、
# 剂型与用法

中药剂量是指临床医师采取的一般用量，尽管中药相对安全，安全剂量的范围也较大，用量不似西药那般严格，但是药物的用量会极大地影响临床疗效。如果用量过小，则达不到治疗效果，同样药物用量过大也会损伤人体的正气，并造成中药资源的浪费，因此合理选择药物剂量是中药应用实践过程中的关键所在。一般而言，同类药物入丸散剂的用量要小于入汤剂的量，而在一张药方中，作为主要治疗作用的君药要比辅助药物的用量大。

中药的用法主要包括中药的给药途径、煎煮方法和服药方法。中药的给药途径范围较广，除常规口服及外用（皮肤给药）的方法外，一般还包括舌下给药、直肠给药、黏膜给药等方式，随着现代制药工艺的发展，目前还衍生出肌内注射、皮下注射、静脉注射、穴位注射等多种给药途径。中药煎煮方法主要为：先将所需煎煮的中药饮片浸泡 30~90 分钟，以便在煎煮时充分发挥中药药效，用水量一般以高出中药材表面为度。煎煮一般分两次进行，第一煎为常规煎，第二煎所加水量为第一煎的1/2左右。两次煎液去渣混合后分早晚2次服用。煎煮火候和时间要依照药物性能确定。一般而言，走表、清热药宜大火快煎，要严格控制煎煮时间，煮沸后煎 3~5 分钟即可，否则会使药物功效降低；偏于补益的中药需小火慢熬，煮沸后需再煎 30~60 分钟，使有效成分得以充分释放。中药的常规服用方式一般为每日 1 剂，分两次服用。服用中药时，一般应温服。服用中药要与饮食间隔至少 30 分钟左右，以免食物的消化吸收影响中药药效的发挥。此外，依据病变部位的不同，服药方法亦各异，病在胸膈以上者，如治疗头痛、眩晕、眼疾、鼻塞、咽痛等药物宜饭后服用；病在胸膈以下者，如治疗脾胃、肝、肾等脏腑疾病的中药，则宜饭前服。因饭前服用中药，可充分发挥药效，便于药物的消化吸收，故多数药都宜饭前服用，但在某些情况下，如个别中药对消化道有刺激者宜饭后服用。

# 第七节
## 中药的应用

## 一、对中药"毒性"的理解

对于中药是不是"毒"药这一问题，古今医家都有不同的见解，但基于中医学原创思维，从宏观的角度去看待和认识中药的毒性，我们可以将这一毒性看作中药治疗疾病的偏性。明代著名医家张景岳在《类经》中谈到："药以治病，因毒为能，所谓毒者，以气味之有偏也。盖气味之正者，谷食之属是也，所以养人之正气。气味之偏者，药饵之属是也，所以去人之邪气，其为故也，正以人之为病，病在阴阳偏胜耳……是凡可辟邪安正者，均可称为毒药，故曰毒药攻邪也。"正是因为中药具有偏性，其才能调节人体的偏性，具体可概括为"以偏纠偏"。由此观之，中药"毒"的概念主要体现其偏性的概念，而真正意义上的毒性则是指我们今天所言的肝肾毒性或其他脏腑毒性。目前中国已经对有毒中药的使用进行了严格的管理，国务院印发了《医疗用毒性药品管理办法》，指出毒性中药包括砒石、砒霜、水银、生马钱子、生川乌、生草乌、生白附子、生附子、生半夏、生南星、生巴豆、斑蝥、青娘虫、红娘虫、生甘遂、生狼毒、生藤黄、生千金子、生天仙子、闹羊花、雪上一枝蒿、红升丹、白降丹、蟾酥、洋金花、红粉、轻粉、雄黄。因此需甄别毒性与偏性的概念，不可混淆。

## 二、中药与药食同源

中国药食同源的历史悠久，许多中医典籍中都记载了与中医食疗调护有关的内容，药食同源类物质本身可以作为实用性的中药材，同时也兼具食养的功能并广泛应用于医疗保健领域。中药中一部分药性相对平淡、偏性不强的中药可作为食养产品的重要来源，如我们所熟知百合、薄荷、枸杞子、菊花、阿胶、山药、薏苡仁、玫瑰花、蜂蜜、荷叶、黑芝麻、马齿苋、蒲公英、莲子、姜、枣等皆是生活中常见的药食同源物质。中医不仅着眼于食物的营养，更注重食物的性味归经。中医理论认为药物具有寒热温凉四气，辛甘酸苦咸五味，同时在经络上，药物有各自的经络归属，食物亦不例外。因此，必须根据体质的寒热虚实辨证使用。根据食物的性质，凡用于治疗热证的食物，大多具有寒凉药性；治疗寒证的食物，大多具有温热药性。根据五味可以确定食物的药效，即酸收、苦降、甘补、辛散、咸软。凡酸味食物多具有收敛、生津、止泻的药效；凡苦味食物多具有清热、泻火、解毒的药效；凡甘味食物多具有濡养、润肠的药效；凡辛味食物多具有解表、行气的药效；凡咸味食物多具软坚、散结、化瘀的药效。因此，中医又根据五味所主的食物归经和药效关系而辨证施膳。一般规律为：辛入肺，甘入脾，酸入肝，苦入心，咸入肾。

# 第八节
## 中药和西药的差异

中药成分复杂，一味中药含有数种甚至数百种化学成分，古人认识中药往往基于哲学思维，对中药的应用也来自临床经验而非实验室指标，因此中药功效的发挥是具有整体性的。西药成分相对单一，药理作用较为明确。我们基于中医学思维视角去正确看待中药和西药，二者在临床诊疗方面往往殊途同归。西医认为细胞突变是疾病的重要成因，包括细胞的功能低下和细胞功能的亢进。对于细胞功能低下者，中医常应用具有扶助正气功效的中药，补气、养血、滋阴、养阳；对于细胞功能亢进者，则常应用具有祛邪解毒功效的中药，以祛除人体不应存在的痰饮、瘀血等病理产物，调节人体的形神合一平衡、气机升降出入平衡、阴阳平衡等。因此我们既要辩证地看待中药与西药的差异，同时尽可能在差异中找出二者的共性，以便更好地指导临床实践。

# 第九节
## 中药在国家医疗体系中的地位

## 一、中药相关的中国政策解读

2017 年 7 月 1 日，《中华人民共和国中医药法》（以下简称为《中医药法》）正式实施。《中医药法》是中国中医药界首部纲领性、标准性、基础性的法律，对规范中医药诊疗行为具有重要意义。它首次从国家法律角度上明确了中医药的重要地位、发展方针和扶持措施，为中医药事业发展提供了法律保障，同时也为中医药行业未来的发展奠定了法制基础。《中医药法》共计 9 章 63 条，其内容涵盖中医药服务、中药保护与发展、中医药人才培养、中医药科学研究、中医药传承与文化传播、保障措施以及法律责任等涉及中医药发展诸多层面的内容。与中药最为相关的国家政策性规范文件是《中华人民共和国药典》（以下简称《中国药典》），其是中国药品标准的最关键的组成部分，也是新药研制、生产、经营、应用和监管等涉及中药应用过程必须遵循的一项法典。国家药典委员会每 5 年组织专家对《中国药典》进行修订，结合临床最新研究对已有内容进行适度更新。现行版为《中国药典》2020 年版，分为 4 部，其中第一部主要收载中药，第二部收载化学药品，第三部收载生物制品，第四部则收载通用技术要求和药用辅料。《中国药典》将中药摆在第一部的核心位置也阐明了中药在中国药品应用领域的重要地位。此外，近年来中国政府还不断发布有利于中药产业发展的文件，如在 2021 年 1 月，国务院办公厅印发《关于加快中医药特色发展的若干政策措施》，明确提出要提高中药产业活力、增强中医药发展活力等。此类文件的发布聚焦中医药发展的困局与难题，体现了中国政府对中医药的政策支持力度与投入力度。

## 二、世界各国对中药的政策

美国于 1994 年颁布《膳食补充剂健康和教育法》，这是一项美国联邦法律，其对膳食补充剂进行了定义，并发布了安全性和有效性声明。其对膳食补充剂的定义包括 "草药或其他植物" 以及其 "任何浓缩物"，这确定了植物提取物作为膳食补充剂的合法地位。

德国对中药的管理有一定的体系性，如在立法程序上允许植物提取物作为处方药进行注册，这在一定程度上肯定了中药的作用。德国注册药品中约有 60 000 种含有草药成分，大部分是草药浸剂，这些药品基于 600~700 种植物，制作的提取物或制剂约 5 000 种。但德国对中药的审核较为严格，如一种中药想要以植物药的身份进入德国，则需要经过复杂的审批程序。保证农残、重金属、微生物含量不超标，质量达到一定要求的药品才可进入德国市场售卖。目前中国中药多以保健品形式进入德国，在程序上按食品管理形式申请。

　　日本虽历史上深受中国文化的影响，是中国中药出口的第一大市场，但汉方药的使用也受到极大的限制。目前除已批准的 210 种方剂外，日本厚生劳动省对新增汉方药的审批异常严格，以等同于化合物新药的方法对待汉方药，并对进口中成药的审批也有不少限制性措施。但近年来，日本政府对健康食品的管制明显趋于缓和，如取消了剂型的限制，放宽了可以用于健康食品的天然植物药种类的限制等。日本推出新的《药事法》，基本的原则是"规制缓和"，对药品生产、流通的管理办法进一步向欧美靠拢，将放松以往严格的限制。

第二章

常用中药

使用指导

# 第一节
## 药食同源中药

## 一、百合

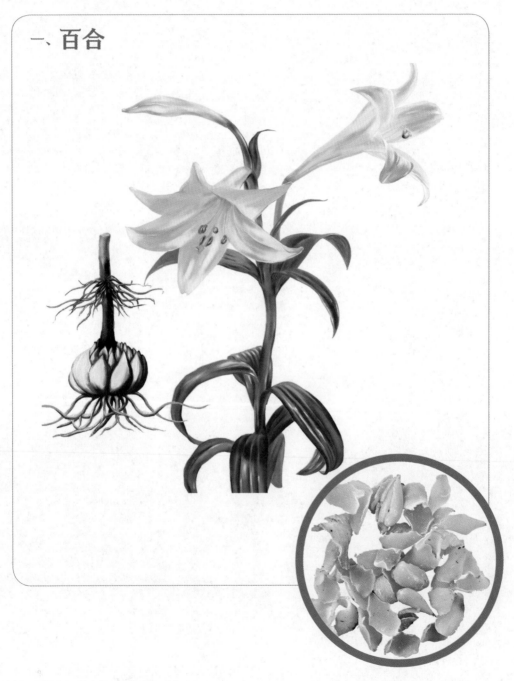

◎ 百合入药用什么?

　　以百合科植物百合、卷丹、细叶百合的肉质鳞叶入药。

◎ 哪里产的百合好?

　　湖南产的百合质量较优。

◎ 如何辨别百合质量的好坏?

　　以瓣匀而肉厚、外表颜色黄白、质坚而筋少、味较苦者为佳。

◎ 百合如何保存?

　　百合喜温怕冷,不耐风吹,受风后其鳞片易变红、干萎。鲜百合清水冲洗去黏液,薄摊晒干或炕干保存,若要鲜用可将百合埋藏在细沙中贮藏,贮藏温度以5~11℃为宜;干百合在干燥阴凉处保存即可。

◎ 百合生用和蜜炙用有什么区别?

　　百合饮片分为生百合和蜜炙百合,前者清心安神效果好,后者养阴润肺效果好。

【广医医师说功效】

◎ **药性与功效——养阴、润肺、清心**

　　百合味甘,性微寒,归肺、心经,具有补益作用。其颜色偏白,中医认为色白主要入肺经,故能养阴润肺;其药性微寒,能够清心、肺、胃经的虚火,有良好的清心安神作用。此外,本品还兼有一定的止咳祛痰作用,外用可以治疗皮肤痈肿和湿疹。

◎ **适用人群——阴虚体质,咽干久咳、虚烦失眠**

　　百合主要适用于心、肺、胃阴虚内热的人群,多用于体形偏瘦、平素怕热、容易盗汗、口干想喝凉水、大便偏干、小便量少偏黄者。

阴虚肺燥为主者，多见干咳少痰、咳血、咽干、嘶哑、烦热、盗汗等。

虚热扰心为主者，多见失眠、心悸、神志恍惚、情绪不能自主、口苦、小便黄等。

阴虚胃热为主者，多见口干唇燥、嘈杂、干呕、饮食减少、食后胸膈不适、大便干结等。

◎ 适用病证

百合可用于肺结核、高热等病症恢复期，神经症，更年期综合征，肺癌中晚期，慢性胃炎，十二指肠溃疡，胃癌中晚期等疾病见阴虚肺燥、虚热扰心、阴虚胃热证候者的治疗。

◎ 什么样的人不适合用百合？

因为百合性质略偏寒凉，而且有养阴敛肺作用，因此外感风寒咳嗽、平素怕冷喜暖、胃寒喜饮热水、大便溏薄者不适合服用百合。

若服用百合后出现怕冷、胃寒、腹泻者应该停用，可适当服用生姜水缓解症状。

【 广医专家话食疗 】

◎ 百合食疗用法用量

百合药性甘润和缓，日常代茶饮可以用 5~15g。居家佐餐如炒菜、煲汤、煮粥等，饮片可以用 10~30g，鲜百合可以用 30~60g。

◎ 百合最适合什么季节服用？

百合四季皆可服用，因为其具有养阴清心的作用，所以尤其适合于夏、秋季节服用。

◎ 如何搭配药材、食材？

百合甘寒滋润，取其养阴疗效时，尤其是滋补肺阴时常佐入白砂糖或蜂蜜等增强其养阴润燥的功效；治疗肺阴不足，干咳少痰或痰中带血，手脚心烦热，盗汗等，常与生地黄、玉竹、麦冬、贝母等合用。

在日常炒菜时常与西芹、苦瓜、竹笋等清热利水的食材搭配，起到清热养阴的功效；煮粥时常可搭配绿豆、薏苡仁等清热健脾；煲汤时常可搭配乌鸡、玉竹、枸杞子等滋阴润燥。

◎ 百合、玉竹食疗时如何选择？

百合与玉竹都是甘寒之品，都具有清肺养阴、清热生津的食疗功效，常搭配使用，可互相提高疗效。百合还能清心安神，因此如有虚烦失眠、心慌多梦选用百合更为适宜。

## 小验方

1. 治疗慢性嗳气、腹胀反复发作

   鲜百合 30g，乌药 9g。煲汤，每日早、晚各 1 次温服。

2. 治疗失眠、神经衰弱

   鲜百合 60g，蜂蜜适量。拌和，蒸熟，睡前服。

3. 治疗溃疡创口不愈

   取鲜百合 100g，冰片少许。同捣烂，拌匀于局部外敷，每日 1 次。

## 二、薄荷

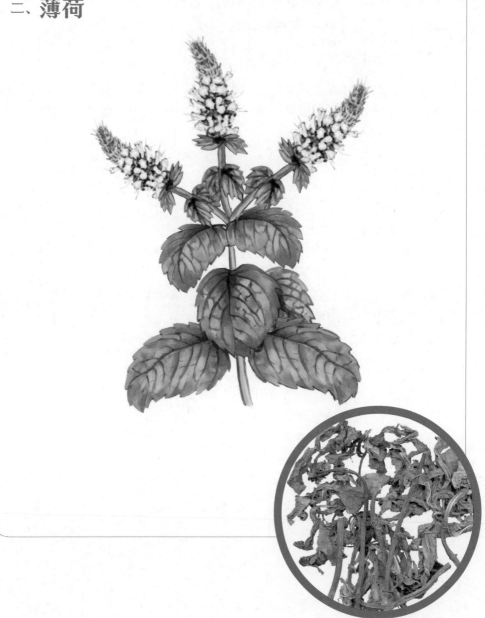

◎ 薄荷入药用什么？

薄荷为唇形科植物薄荷的干燥地上部分。

◎ 哪里产的薄荷好？

江苏苏州地区产量大而质优。

◎ 如何辨别薄荷质量的好坏？

以叶多、色深绿、味清凉、香气浓者为佳，一般认为江苏太仓的栽培头刀薄荷质优。

◎ 薄荷如何保存？

鲜薄荷多于割后摊晒干或阴干保存。干薄荷阴凉处保存即可。

◎ 薄荷叶与薄荷梗功用有什么区别？

薄荷叶发汗解表的功效较好，薄荷梗偏于行气和中。

【广医医师说功效】

◎ 药性与功效——疏散风热，清利头目，利咽透疹，疏肝解郁

薄荷性凉味辛，辛以发散，凉以清热，归于肺经，具有疏散风热作用；其颜色为绿色，中医认为色苍主要入肝经，其性辛散，故能疏肝解郁。此外，本品还兼有一定的辟秽气作用，可用于治疗暑湿吐泻。

◎ 适用人群——外感风热，头痛目赤、胸闷胁痛

薄荷主要适用于外感风热之邪的人群，多用于体质壮实之人风热感冒，症见发热、微恶风寒、咽干口渴、头痛目赤等。

本品能疏肝行气，治疗肝气郁滞之人，多见胸胁胀痛、月经不调等。

◎ 适用病证

薄荷可用于治疗风热感冒、头痛、咽喉痛、口舌生疮、风疹、麻疹、胸腹胀闷等。另外，薄荷还具有消炎止痛作用。

◎ 什么样的人不适合用薄荷？

因为薄荷性寒凉，芳香辛散、发汗耗气，故体虚多汗、脾虚便溏者不宜使用。孕妇、产妇及幼儿应避免食用。

薄荷毒副作用很少见，误服薄荷油可能出现头昏、眼花、恶心、呕吐、手足麻木、逐渐昏迷、血压略降。

【 广医专家话食疗 】

◎ 薄荷食疗用法用量

薄荷茎叶有特殊的清凉香味，疏散风热、清利头目、利咽、透疹、疏肝解郁，日常代茶饮可以用 5~15g。居家佐餐如薄荷糕、薄荷汤、薄荷粥，饮片可以用 15g，鲜薄荷可以用 30g。但因薄荷含有芳香性挥发油，泡茶时应加盖为好，无论泡茶还是煎汤时间都不宜过久，一般 5~6 分钟即可。

◎ 薄荷最适合什么季节服用？

薄荷四季皆可服用，因其具有疏散风热、辟秽化浊的功效，尤其适合于春、夏季服用。

◎ 如何搭配药材、食材？

薄荷辛凉，用其疏散风热时多配伍金银花、连翘、牛蒡子、荆芥等。若用于肝气郁滞，胸胁闷痛，常与柴胡、白芍、当归等合用。

在日常煮粥时薄荷可搭配绿豆、薏苡仁等清热健脾；与绿豆、糯米制成糕点以清热疏风；炒菜时可与豆腐、鸡丝等搭配以清热。

## 小验方

1. **治疗肺热所导致的咳嗽、咽痛**

   薄荷 10g,橄榄 50g,萝卜 100g。三者同放入锅中,加水煎煮后取药汁服用。

2. **治疗痰气阻滞所致耳鸣、耳聋**

   陈皮、芦根各 10g,荸荠 3 个,薄荷 6g。将除薄荷外的原料洗净放入锅中,加水煮汤,最后放入薄荷略煮后关火,取汁代茶饮用。

# 三、枸杞子

第二章 常用中药使用指导

【广医药师谈选药】

◎ 哪里产的枸杞子好？

　　宁夏、甘肃、青海出产的枸杞子质量较优。

◎ 如何辨别枸杞子质量的好坏？

　　以粒大、色红、肉厚、籽少、质柔润、味甜者为佳。

◎ 枸杞子如何保存？

　　枸杞子含糖较多，极易吸潮泛油、发霉或虫蛀，而且容易变色。置于冰箱中 0~4℃保存，是简单、实用的一种贮藏方法。

【广医医师说功效】

◎ 药性与功效——滋肾、补肝、明目、润肺

　　枸杞子性味甘平，具有补益作用，擅滋补肝肾之阴，中医认为肝开窍于目，目精属肾，肝肾阴足则目自明，故其能明目；通过滋补肝肾之阴，具有养血之功，能治面色萎黄；能生津止渴，同时又能兼入肺经滋阴润肺。

◎ 适用人群——阴虚体质，咽干久咳、虚烦失眠

　　枸杞子性质平和，无明显偏性，其效力较缓和，无妨碍消化之弊，体质虚弱的人可以久服常用。主要适用于肝肾阴精、阴血亏虚的人群，多用于体形偏瘦、面色暗黄，腰酸腿软，失眠多梦，头发、胡须早白，牙齿松动者。

　　肝肾阴虚，不能制阳为主者，多见头晕目眩、腰腿酸软、视物昏花等。

　　肝肾不足，阴血亏虚者，多见失眠、多梦、面色萎黄等。

　　内热伤阴为主者，多见口干唇燥、嘈杂、干呕、饮食减少、食后胸膈不适、大便干结等。

◎ 适用病证

枸杞子可用于贫血、慢性疲劳综合征、化学性肝损伤、糖尿病、高脂血症、高血压、肿瘤、慢性萎缩性胃炎、不育症等疾病见肝肾阴虚、阴血亏虚证候者的治疗。

◎ 什么样的人不适合用枸杞子?

枸杞子虽然滋腻性较小,但毕竟是味甘质润之品,因此有脾胃虚弱,大便溏薄,平素怕冷喜暖、胃寒喜饮热水者应少用枸杞子。

【 广医专家话食疗 】

◎ 枸杞子食疗用法用量

枸杞子药性甘润和缓,日常代茶饮可以用 5~10g。居家佐餐如炒菜、煲汤、煮粥等,饮片可以用 5~15g,鲜枸杞子可以用 10~30g。

◎ 枸杞子最适合什么季节服用?

枸杞子四季皆可服用,因为其具有滋补肝肾的作用,所以尤其适合于秋、冬季节服用。

◎ 如何搭配药材、食材?

枸杞子甘平,取其滋补肝肾疗效时,尤其是养肝明目时常佐入熟地黄、菊花等增强其滋阴明目的功效;治疗阴血亏虚,面色萎黄,可与鸡蛋同煮,吃蛋喝汤,伴有失眠多梦者也可与龙眼肉等合用。

在日常煮粥时常与山药、薏苡仁等益气健脾的食材搭配;煲汤时常可搭配乌鸡、玉竹、百合等滋阴润燥。

◎ 枸杞子、桑椹食疗时如何选择?

桑椹性质甘寒,具有滋阴补血、生津、润肠的食疗功效,可与枸杞子搭配使用,以增强补肝肾、益阴血的功效。桑椹还能润肠,因此如有血虚肠燥便秘、内热口渴表现者选用桑椹更为适宜。

**小验方**

1. 治疗不育症

   每晚嚼食枸杞子 15g，连服 1 个月为一疗程。

2. 治疗慢性萎缩性胃炎

   枸杞子每日 20g，分两次空腹时嚼服，2 个月为一疗程。

3. 治疗头晕、目眩、耳鸣

   取枸杞子 30~60g，每日水煎，频服。

# 四、金银花

◎ 金银花有几种，哪种更好？

　　金银花按产区分为密银花、济银花，以河南出产的密银花品质优。

◎ 如何辨别金银花质量的好坏？

　　以花蕾初开、完整、色黄白、无杂质者为佳。

◎ 金银花如何保存？

　　鲜品宜放在阴凉处晾干，于干燥通风处存放。

◎ 金银花生用、炒炭和制露剂功效有什么区别？

　　金银花可生用、炒炭用，还可以用蒸汽蒸馏法制成金银花露。生用发散风热，尤其是清里热效果好；炒炭后清透之功已失，凉血解毒止痢效果好；金银花露则具有清热解暑的功效。

【广医医师说功效】

◎ 药性与功效——清热解毒、疏散风热、凉血止痢

　　中医认为金银花质轻，有疏散风热的作用。金银花性味甘寒，归肺、心、胃经，能够清热解毒。其气味芳香，还可解血中之毒。

◎ 适用人群——肺热体质，咽喉肿痛，疮痈疔疖，热毒泻痢

　　金银花主要适用于肺热体质的人群。多用于平素耐冷、外感风热咽喉肿痛、发热、汗出、口渴、疮痈肿毒、大便下痢脓血者。

　　外感风热为主者，多见发热、头痛、咽痛、口渴等。

　　疮痈疔疖者，多见局部红肿热痛，成脓甚至破溃等。

　　热毒泻痢为主者，多见下痢脓血、肠鸣腹痛，大便不爽、肛门灼热等。

◎ 适用病证

金银花可用于温病发热、热毒血痢、痈肿疔疮及多种感染性疾病的治疗。

◎ 什么样的人不适合用金银花？

因为金银花性质寒凉，因此体质虚弱，食欲不振，平素怕冷喜暖、大便稀溏，脾胃虚寒者慎服。正气不足，平素所生疮疡流脓透亮清稀的人群也不适宜服用。

若服用金银花后出现怕冷、胃寒、大便溏泄者应该停用，可适当服用桂皮等缓解症状。

【 广医专家话食疗 】

◎ 金银花食疗用法用量

金银花药性甘寒，日常代茶饮可以用 5~10g。

◎ 金银花最适合什么季节服用？

金银花四季皆可服用。因为其具有清热解毒的作用，所以尤其适合于夏季服用。

◎ 如何搭配药材、食材？

金银花甘寒质轻，取其透散表邪，治疗风热感冒时，常常搭配荆芥、薄荷、连翘等；对于生疮痈疔疖者，常与蒲公英、野菊花、黄芩等合用；用于治疗热毒下痢脓血者，可配合黄连、黄芩、白头翁等增强清热凉血止痢的效果。

可与粳米搭配制成金银花粥，清热解暑；与荷叶、菊花等制成凉茶，可预防中暑、感冒及肠道传染病等。

◎ 金银花、忍冬藤食疗时如何选择？

金银花与忍冬藤功用相似，都具有清热解毒、疏散风热等食疗功效。忍冬藤疏散风热表邪作用不如金银花，但有通络止痛的作用，内服可治疗关节红肿热痛，屈伸不利等。

1. **治疗热毒疮疡**

   忍冬藤、黄芪、甘草以 2∶4∶1 比例，切细，酒浸，煎服。

2. **治疗热毒痢疾**

   忍冬藤 100~200g，浓煎饮服。

# 五、菊花

◎ 哪里产的菊花好？

  以安徽亳州、河南商丘产的亳菊，以及安徽滁州产的滁菊质量较优。

◎ 如何辨别菊花质量的好坏？

  菊花均以身干、色白（黄）、花朵完整不散瓣、香气浓郁、无杂质者为佳。

◎ 菊花如何保存？

  需放置在阴凉干燥的环境下贮存，避免潮湿。

◎ 黄菊花和白菊花功效有什么不同？

  疏散风热多用黄菊花（杭菊），平肝明目用白菊花（滁菊）。

【广医医师说功效】

◎ 药性与功效——疏风、平肝、清热、明目

  菊花味辛、质地轻盈，中医认为辛味的中药能够行散气血，上达头面，外达肌表，故能疏风；其性微寒，中医认为性寒的中药能够清热，因此本品能够疏风清热；本品入肺经，能够治疗风热犯肺引起的发热、咽痛、咳嗽等症；本品亦入肝经，疏散风热的同时又能平抑肝阳，从而治疗肝阳上亢引起的头痛、眩晕，亦可清泻肝火、明目退翳，治疗肝火上炎引起的目赤肿痛等。

◎ 适用人群——湿热体质，风热犯肺、肝阳上亢、肝火上炎

  菊花主要适用于湿热体质的人群，多用于性情急躁、平素怕热、感冒后易发热咽痛、容易出汗、口干想喝凉水、大便偏干、小便偏黄者。

  风热犯肺为主者，感冒后多见发热重、微恶风、头胀痛、咽喉红肿疼痛、咳嗽、痰黏或黄、鼻塞黄涕、口渴喜饮等。

  肝阳上亢为主者，多见急躁易怒、头晕、头痛等。

肝火上炎为主者，多见目赤肿痛、面部疔疮等。

◎ 适用病证

菊花可用于感冒发热，咽炎、高血压、结膜炎等疾病见风热犯肺、肝阳上亢、肝火上炎证候者的治疗。

◎ 什么样的人不适合用菊花？

菊花性质略偏寒凉，因此外感风寒咳嗽，头痛而恶寒，平素怕冷喜暖、胃寒喜饮热水、大便溏薄者不适合服用菊花。

若服用菊花后出现怕冷、胃寒、腹泻者应该停用，可适当服用生姜水缓解症状。

【 广医专家话食疗 】

◎ 菊花食疗用法用量

菊花药性微寒和缓，食疗最宜日常代茶饮，可以用 3~5g。

◎ 菊花最适合什么季节服用？

菊花四季皆可服用，因为其具有疏风清热的功效，所以尤其适合于春、夏季节服用。

◎ 如何搭配药材、食材？

取其疏风清热疗效时，常配薄荷、金银花、桑叶等，沸水浸泡，代茶饮；取其平抑肝阳功效时，常配天麻、钩藤等，沸水浸泡，代茶饮；取其清肝泄热、明目功效时，常用决明子、枸杞子、夏枯草、谷精草等，沸水浸泡，代茶饮。

◎ 菊花、野菊花食疗时如何选择？

菊花与野菊花都是味辛、微寒之品，都具有疏风清热的食疗功效，常搭配使用，可互相提高疗效，但野菊花清热解毒之力更强，因此如有颜面疔疮、疖肿者选用野菊花更为适宜。

## 小验方

1. 治疗感冒发热，头昏，目赤，咽喉不利

    菊花6g，薄荷9g，金银花、桑叶各10g。沸水浸泡，代茶饮。

2. 防治早期高血压

    菊花10g，茶叶3g。沸水浸泡，代茶饮。

3. 治疗肝热目赤、头晕目眩

    菊花10g，炒决明子12g。沸水浸泡，代茶饮。

## 六、阿胶

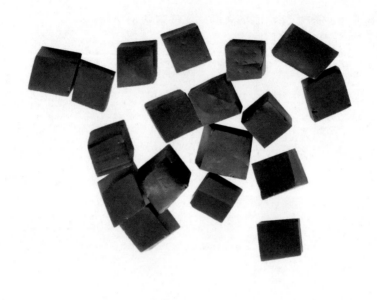

【广医药师谈选药】

◎ 如何辨别阿胶的真伪?

阿胶当以黄透如琥珀色,光黑如漆者为真。真者无皮臭味,夏日亦不湿软。手持用力拍打桌面,碎片断面呈棕色、半透明、无异物者为真,若拍打软而不碎者,则疑为伪品。

◎ 阿胶如何保存?

阿胶长久风吹则易干裂破碎,日晒则易发软,受潮、受热则易回潮变软。其安全水分含量为 16%~18%,含水量超过 21% 则开始生霉,相对湿度在 75% 以下,则水分散失,胶面脆裂。故贮藏的适宜相对湿度以 80%~85% 为宜,若吸湿过多,可用石灰、氯化钙等干燥。当夏季空气湿热时,宜贮于冰箱内。

◎ 阿胶与龟甲胶、鹿角胶有什么区别？

龟甲胶表面棕色略带微绿，上面有黄色"油头"，对光视之洁净如琥珀，质坚硬；鹿角胶表面黑棕色，对光视之半透明，一面有黄白色多孔性薄层，质脆易碎，断面红棕色，具玻璃光泽。

## 【广医医师说功效】

◎ 药性与功效——补血，滋阴，润肺，止血

阿胶味甘，中医认为甘味的中药具有补益的作用，其为血肉有情之品，为补血要约；中医认为阿胶可以入肺、肝、肾经而滋补阴血，因此该药还有滋阴润肺、滋补肝肾的作用。另外本品质黏，可用于止血。

◎ 适用人群——阴血两虚之人，出血证

阿胶主要适用于阴血两虚的人群，尤其是肺、肝、肾阴血两虚的患者。多用于阴虚血热吐衄，血虚、虚寒之崩漏下血，心悸，咳嗽痰少，咽喉干燥，痰中带血，心烦不得眠者。

肺热阴虚为主者，多见咳嗽痰少、咽喉干燥、痰中带血等。

肾阴虚、心火亢者，多见心烦、不欲寐等。

◎ 适用病证

阿胶擅于治疗血虚引起的各种病症，并通过补血起到滋润皮肤的作用，还能调经保胎，增强体质，改善睡眠，健脑益智，延缓衰老，亦可用于神经衰弱、头昏、失眠多梦、神疲乏力等症的治疗。

◎ 什么样的人不适合用阿胶？

因阿胶味甘质黏，凡脾胃虚弱，呕吐泄泻，腹胀便溏、咳嗽痰多者慎用。感冒患者不宜服用。孕妇、高血压、糖尿病患者应在医师指导下服用。小儿应在医师指导下服用。女性行经期间慎用，或在医师指导下使用。孕妇保胎需在医师指导下使用。阴虚阳亢体质的人群，需要酌情减量或者减少频率使用，以防出现喉痛等上火症状。阴虚阳亢体质具体症状表现为：晨起口干舌燥、眼屎多、大便干、易急躁。

◎ 阿胶食疗用法用量

阿胶药性甘平，日常可完全融化后冷藏，每日温开水冲服。居家佐餐如煲汤、煮粥等，可以用 5~10g。

◎ 阿胶最适合什么季节服用？

阿胶四季皆可服用，冬末春初，人体一身气血经过一冬的蛰伏，在此时转为升发，所以正是进补的最佳时机。这个时候服用阿胶，往往能对阳气的振奋起到很好的作用。

◎ 如何搭配药材、食材？

阿胶甘平，取其补血止血，治疗出血而致血虚者为佳，常搭配熟地黄、当归、芍药等；治疗肺阴虚咳嗽者，常搭配牛蒡子、苦杏仁等。

煮粥时常可搭配冰糖等补血益肾；煲汤时常可搭配雪梨、冰糖、鸡蛋等润肺止咳。

**小验方**

**治疗肺燥咳嗽、久病多痰**

雪梨 1~2 个，切成小块后加水煮沸，然后加入阿胶小碎块 12g，用筷子反复搅拌使之溶化，加入白糖或冰糖 50g，蜂蜜 50g。喝汤吃梨。

# 七、山药

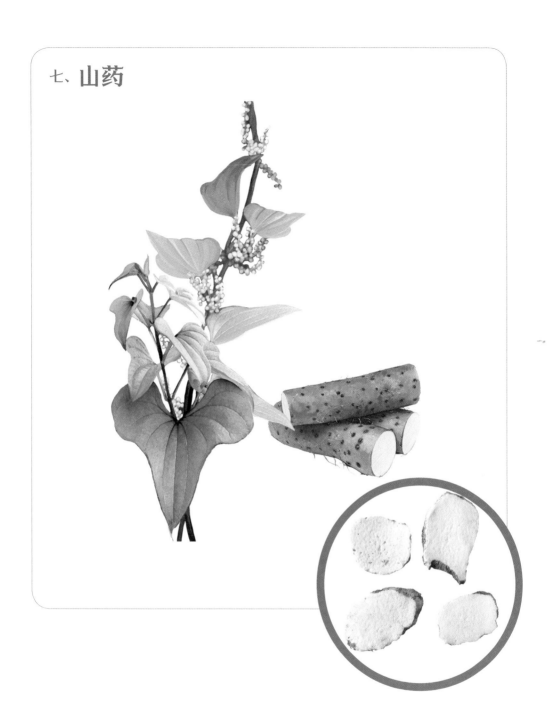

◎ 山药入药用什么？

以薯蓣科植物薯蓣的根茎入药，生用或麸炒用。

◎ 哪里产的山药最好？

山药以河南怀庆所产为佳，故有"怀山药"之名。

◎ 如何辨别山药质量的好坏？

以根块大，果肉黏液多（掰断可看出有黏液），根须多，外皮无损伤，断层雪白，水分少者为佳。

◎ 山药如何保存？

山药耐寒，必要时可以就地贮存。山药块茎休眠期较耐低温，适宜的贮藏温度为 0~2℃，相对湿度 90% 左右。常用的贮藏方法为筐藏法：把日晒消毒的稻草或麦草铺垫在消过毒的筐或箱四周。然后把选好的山药逐层堆至八分满，上面用麦草覆盖。最后堆放在库房内，保持库内适温，为防止地面湿气，可在筐底垫上砖头或木板。

◎ 山药生用和麸炒用有什么区别？

山药饮片分为生山药和麸炒山药，前者补肾固精效果好，后者补肺益气效果好。

【 广医医师说功效 】

◎ **药性与功效——补脾养胃，生津益肺，补肾涩精**

山药味甘，具有补益作用，入肺、脾、肾经；性平，能够益气养阴，补脾肺肾，固精止带。由于其气阴双补的特点，对以气阴两虚为主要病机的糖尿病患者也有一定疗效。

◎ **适用人群——脾虚湿盛，肺虚咳喘，肾虚滑精**

山药主要适用于肺、脾、肾三脏气阴两虚的人群，多用于平素乏力、食少、大便稀溏、夜尿频多或遗尿，久病咳喘，女子带下量多清稀，男子遗精、滑精、早泄者。

脾气虚为主者，多见消瘦或肥胖乏力、食少、腹胀、大便稀溏，女子带下量多等。

肺气虚为主者，多见咳喘无力、气短、咳痰色白清稀、自汗怕风、易感冒等。

肾气虚为主者，多见腰膝酸软、耳鸣、耳聋、神疲、乏力、尿频、遗尿、夜尿多，男子滑精、早泄等。

◎ 适用病证

山药可用于慢性胃炎、慢性肾炎、长期腹泻、早泄，以及各种慢性病日久身体虚弱见肺气虚、脾失健运、肾气不足证候的患者。

◎ 什么样的人不适合用山药？

山药有收涩的作用，故平素大便燥结者不宜食用，以防便秘；另外正在处于肾炎、肺炎等疾病急性期的患者忌食山药。

山药与甘遂不要一同食用；也不可与碱性药物同服。

【广医专家话食疗】

◎ 山药食疗用法用量

山药药性甘润和缓，适合各类人群食用。居家佐餐根据炒菜、煲汤、煮粥等不同烹调方法用量不同，饮片可用 10~30g，鲜山药可用 30~60g。

◎ 山药最适合什么季节服用？

山药四季皆可服用，因为其对肺、脾、肾三脏皆有补益作用，不同季节服用各有所长。补肺气可秋季服用，健脾气一年四季皆可，益肾气冬季最佳。

◎ 如何搭配药材、食材？

山药味甘性平，取其补肺气疗效时，与太子参、南沙参等品共奏补肺定喘之效；治疗脾气不足，食少、腹胀、便溏时，与党参、白术等药共用健脾益气；治疗肾虚时，与生地黄、茯苓等药共用补肾利水，历代不少补肾名方如肾气丸、六味地黄丸中均配有本品。

在日常炒菜时常与木耳搭配，既增进食欲，又起到补肾的作用。煮粥时常可搭配芡实、薏苡仁利湿健脾，亦可搭配大枣气血双补，健脾开胃。

◎ 山药、芡实食疗时如何选择？

山药与芡实均为味甘、性平之品，都具有健脾止泻、补肾固精的食疗功效，常搭配使用，可互相提高疗效。与芡实比，山药还能补肺气，养肺阴。因此如有久病虚劳咳喘，气短等症者用山药效果更佳。

**小验方**

1. 治疗脾胃虚弱，饮食减少，消化不良

山药60g，切成小块，大枣30g，粳米适量。加水煮成稀粥，用糖调味服食。

2. 治疗久病咳喘，痰少或无痰，咽干口燥

鲜山药60g，切碎，捣烂，加甘蔗汁半碗和匀，火上炖熟，温服。

3. 治疗遗精、健忘、失眠、羸瘦等

山药50g，芡实50g，粳米50g。加水煮粥，盐调味后即成，每晚温热服食。

# 八、薏苡仁

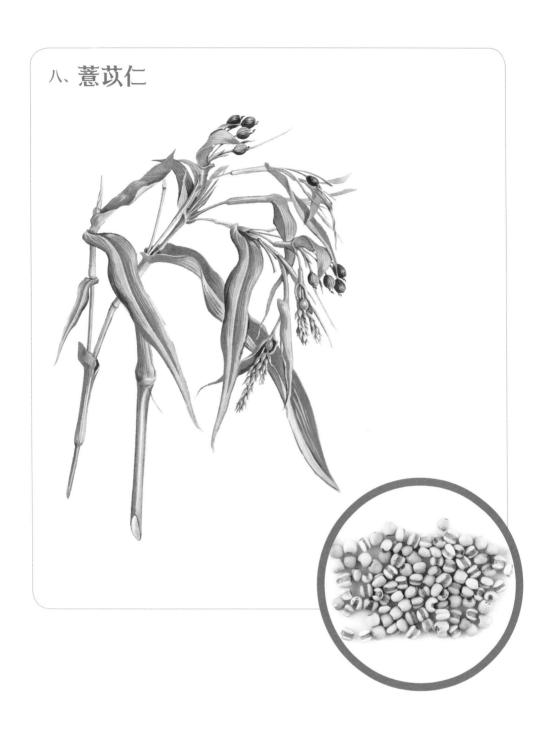

◎ **薏苡仁入药用什么？**

以禾本科植物薏米的干燥成熟种仁入药。

◎ **哪里产的薏苡仁最好？**

中国大部分地区均产，以产于福建、河北、辽宁等地者质优。

◎ **如何辨别薏苡仁质量的好坏？**

以粒大坚实、色白、无皮碎者为佳。

◎ **薏苡仁如何保存？**

薏苡仁喜燥恶湿，在通风、阴凉的干燥处保存，贮温以 5~11℃ 为宜，并注意防止虫蛀。

◎ **薏苡仁生用和麸炒有什么区别？**

薏苡仁饮片分为生薏苡仁和炒薏苡仁，前者清热利湿效果好，后者健脾止泻效果好。

【 广医医师说功效 】

◎ **药性与功效——利水渗湿、健脾、清热排脓、除痹**

薏苡仁味甘、淡，性微凉，归脾、胃、肺经。本品淡渗甘补，既利水消肿，又健脾补中止泻，还可舒筋脉、缓拘挛，清热排脓。可以治疗脾虚湿盛引起的腹泻、肿胀、小便不利及感受风湿之邪引起的关节痹痛。

◎ **适用人群——脾虚痰湿体质，水肿腹胀、筋脉痹痛**

薏苡仁主要适用于脾虚湿盛体质的人群，多用于体形偏胖、平素乏力、小便不利、腹泻、易水肿者，对肺热咳吐脓痰者也有一定疗效。

脾虚湿盛为主者，多见水肿、乏力、困倦、口渴不欲饮水、腹胀、小便不利、腹泻等。

◎ 适用病证

薏苡仁可用于慢性腹泻，风湿性关节炎，慢性阑尾炎，慢性胃炎，中暑，脚气见水肿、脾虚泄泻等证属脾虚湿盛者。

◎ 什么样的人不适合用薏苡仁？

薏苡仁适合各类人群，但因其功以利水渗湿为主，故脾虚无湿、大便干燥、无汗之人以及孕妇慎服。

【广医专家话食疗】

◎ 薏苡仁食疗用法用量

薏苡仁服用方便，超市及药店均可购得，煮粥时以60g左右为宜，熬汤时可用至150g。本品力缓，宜多服久服。

◎ 薏苡仁最适合什么季节服用？

薏苡仁四季皆可服用，因其渗湿利水之功效明显，在夏季及长夏（农历5—8月）暑湿当令之时服用效果最佳。

◎ 如何搭配药材、食材？

薏苡仁渗湿利水，治疗小便不利时常与茯苓、白术、黄芪配伍；治疗脚气浮肿时可与防己、木瓜、苍术同用。此外，本品尤宜治疗脾虚湿盛之泄泻，常与人参、茯苓、白术合用；治疗筋脉挛急疼痛时与独活、防风、苍术配伍。

在煮粥时常可搭配山药、绿豆清热健脾，或与粳米同煮健脾除湿；煲汤时亦可搭配羊肉益气补虚，健脾补肾。

◎ 薏苡仁、茯苓食疗时如何选择？

薏苡仁与茯苓均为利水消肿，渗湿健脾之品。然而茯苓性平补益心脾，宁心安神；薏苡仁性凉而清热，又擅排脓除痹。两者常搭配使用，相辅相成。

**小验方**

1. 治疗脾肺阴虚，饮食懒进，虚热劳嗽，慢性嗳气、腹胀反复发作

   薏苡仁、山药各60g，捣为粗末，加水煮至烂熟。

2. 治疗失眠、神经衰弱、大便秘结，小便短赤等属湿热瘀阻之证

   薏苡仁15g，冬瓜子30g，桃仁10g，牡丹皮6g。加水煎服。

3. 治疗水肿、小便不利，喘息胸满等

   郁李仁60g，研烂，用水滤取药汁；薏苡仁200g，用郁李仁汁煮成饭。每日分2次服。

# 九、玫瑰花

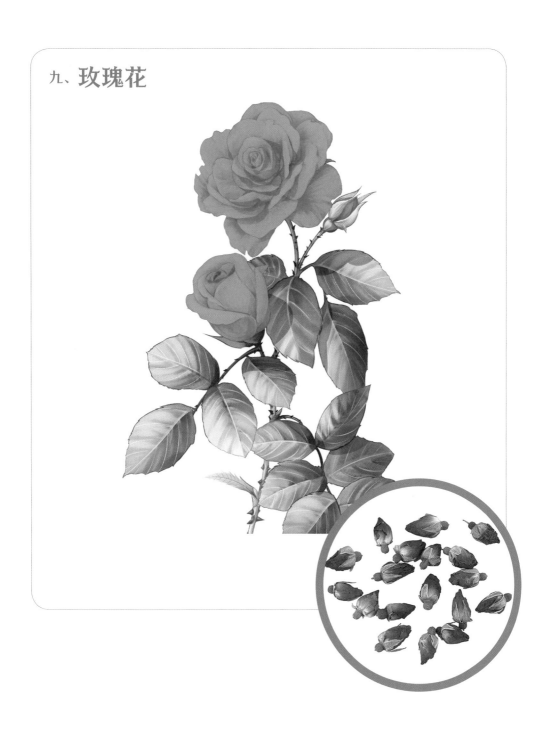

◎ 玫瑰花属于哪一科植物，用药部位是什么？

玫瑰花为蔷薇科植物玫瑰的干燥花蕾。

◎ 玫瑰的产地主要在哪里？

原产地为中国北部地区，全国各地均有庭院栽培，主产于江苏、浙江、福建、山东、四川等地。

◎ 玫瑰花有哪几种颜色？

玫瑰花按颜色主要分为：红玫瑰、黄玫瑰、紫玫瑰、白玫瑰、黑玫瑰、橘红色玫瑰和蓝玫瑰，药用与食用玫瑰花多以红玫瑰与紫玫瑰为主。

◎ 如何采收与保存玫瑰花？

春末、夏初玫瑰花蕾刚开放时采收，采摘已充分膨大但未开放的花蕾，烘干或晒干备用，亦可用鲜品。放于干燥阴凉处保存即可。

◎ 玫瑰花用鲜品与炮制后干品有何区别？

玫瑰花常用的为玫瑰花鲜品与炮制后干品，前者疏肝解郁效果好，后者活血止痛效果好。

◎ 药性与功效——疏肝解郁，活血止痛

玫瑰花味道以甘甜为主，略带苦味，气味芳香，具有理气活血的作用，其颜色紫红，中医认为主要入肝经，能疏肝解郁；其药性微温，又能够活血消肿止痛，有良好的活血止痛作用。此外，本品还兼有一定的芳香醒脾和胃的作用，外用还可以治疗跌打损伤、瘀肿疼痛。

◎ 适用人群——气滞血瘀体质，心情抑郁、月经失调

玫瑰花主要适用于气滞血瘀体质的人群，多用于体形偏瘦、心情抑郁、月经不调、乳房胀痛等。

肝气郁滞为主者，多见心情抑郁、闷闷不乐、唉声叹气、胸胁胀闷不适等。

瘀血阻滞为主者，多见心痛、腹痛、跌打损伤、瘀肿疼痛，女性可见经期乳房胀痛、月经不调、痛经、月经色暗有血块等。

肝气犯胃为主者，多见胸胁脘腹胀闷疼痛、食少、恶心反酸，甚至呕吐等。

◎ 适用病证

玫瑰花可用于治疗抑郁症、乳腺增生、月经不调、痛经、胃痛、消化不良、跌打损伤等见气滞血瘀证者。

◎ 什么样的人不适合用玫瑰花？

玫瑰花性质略偏温热，具有行气活血的作用，比较适合大部分人，尤其是女性，可泡玫瑰花茶喝。由于玫瑰花能够活血行气，所以血热、血虚的患者应少用为宜，出血患者中医辨证不属于气滞血瘀者应禁用。


【广医专家话食疗】


◎ 玫瑰花食疗用法用量

玫瑰花气味芳香，味以甘甜为主，日常代茶饮可以用 3~6g，鲜玫瑰花可以用至 10g，也可直接用玫瑰花蕾 5~10 朵。

◎ 玫瑰花最适合什么季节服用？

玫瑰花四季皆可服用，因为其具有疏肝解郁的作用，尤其适合于春天服用。

◎ 如何搭配药材、食材？

玫瑰花芳香甘温，治疗肝气郁滞，见心情抑郁、闷闷不乐、唉声叹气、

胸胁胀闷不适等时，常常搭配月季花、香附、梅花、郁金、合欢花、柴胡等增强其疏肝解郁的功效；治疗肝气犯胃，见胸胁脘腹胀闷疼痛、食少、恶心反酸，甚至呕吐等时，常与砂仁、山楂、神曲、麦芽、香橼、佛手等合用；治疗瘀血阻滞，见心痛、腹痛、跌打损伤、瘀肿疼痛，女性可见经期乳房胀痛、月经不调、痛经、月经色暗有血块等时，常配合丹参、当归、川芎、三七、泽兰、益母草、鸡冠花等使用。

此外，玫瑰花与冰糖或红糖熬膏，存于瓷瓶密闭保存，早晚各1匙，温开水冲服，可治疗月经不调。鲜玫瑰花适量洗净捣汁，加冰糖炖服可治疗肺病咳血或痰中带血。

◎ 玫瑰花、月季花食疗时如何选择？

玫瑰花与月季花都是理气之品，都具有疏肝解郁、行气活血的食疗功效，常搭配使用，可互相提高疗效。与月季花比，玫瑰花芳香浓郁，理气疏肝解郁的功效较强，因此以心情抑郁、闷闷不乐、唉声叹气、胸胁胀闷不适等为主要表现的肝气郁滞证更为适宜。

## 小验方

1. 治疗胃痛、消化不良、肺病咳血

玫瑰花100g捣碎，与白砂糖300g混匀，置阳光下，待糖溶化后服用。每日3次，每次10g。此膏可以长期食用，具有强身健体，和脾健胃，润肤美容之功。

2. 治疗梅核气，咽中异物感，吐之不出，咽之不下

玫瑰花12g，半夏、大枣、紫苏梗各10g。水煎服，每日1剂。

3. 治疗乳痈，乳房肿痛

玫瑰花7朵，母丁香7粒，加黄酒适量，水煎服。

# 十、蜂蜜

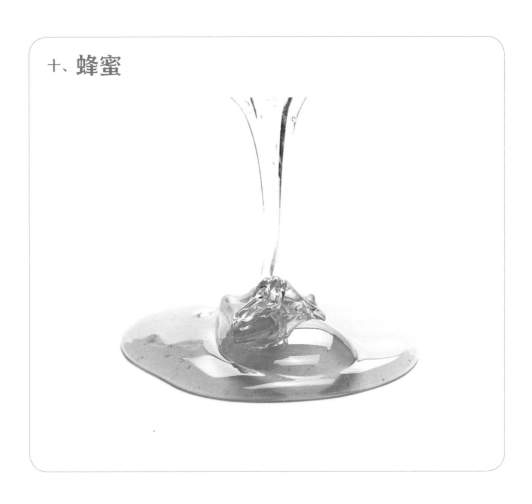

【广医药师谈选药】

◎ 哪里产的蜂蜜质量较好?

以新疆、海南等地产的蜂蜜质量为优。

◎ 如何辨别蜂蜜质量的好坏?

蜂蜜有黄、白之分,古人以白蜜为上品。以色泽清透,光亮如油,质地黏稠,可拉"蜜丝",结晶细腻,甜而微酸,口感绵软细腻者为佳。

◎ 蜂蜜如何保存?

蜂蜜储存怕强光,过强的光照会极大地破坏蜂蜜中的维生素 B 族,导致营养成分流失。保存时应注意将蜂蜜置于低温、避光、干燥、清洁、通风的环境中，贮温以 5~15℃ 为宜，空气湿度不宜超过 75%。

◎ 蜂蜜生用和熟用有什么区别？蜂蜜还有什么其他功效？

蜂蜜生则性凉，故能清热；熟则性温，故能补中。亦因其甘而平和能解毒，因其柔而濡泽能润燥，因其缓可去急能止痛，调和药性，助力其他药物功效的发挥。

## 【 广医医师说功效 】

◎ 药性与功效——补中、润燥、止痛、解毒

蜂蜜味道甘甜，性平和，微温。归脾、肺、胃、大肠经。味甘，可入脾，故能补中健脾。脾气得养，饮食自下，通润肠道。肺喜润而恶燥，蜂蜜润则亦入肺。蜂蜜性平和能缓急止痛，调和诸药，同时亦可协助解毒。

◎ 适用人群——中气不足，阴虚体质，疼痛诸症

蜂蜜主要适用于中气不足，体内津液不足，以及患有疼痛诸症的人群，且多用于便秘人群。

中气不足为主者，多见饮食不佳、纳谷不香、神疲乏力、四肢痿软等。

阴虚为主者，多见潮热盗汗、便秘、干咳、咯血等。

疼痛诸症为主者，多见五脏诸不足引起的疼痛、心腹肌肉疮疡之痛等。

◎ 适用病证

蜂蜜可用于治疗胃痛、便秘、乏力、疼痛等属阴虚证、气虚证者。

◎ 什么样的人不适合用蜂蜜？

蜂蜜味甘则壅，故脾胃虚寒者忌用；体润性滑，故泄泻者忌用。服蜂蜜时不可与生葱同食。若与莴苣同食，令人利下。

◎ 蜂蜜食疗用法用量

蜂蜜味甘性平和，日常可用温水冲服，成人可用25g左右，儿童应控制在10g左右。可以和白萝卜一起煮润肺止咳，和枸杞子一起煮护肝，用10~20g即可。

◎ 蜂蜜最适合什么季节服用？

蜂蜜四季皆可服用。春季服用蜂蜜利于消除疲劳；夏季冷水冲服蜂蜜可消暑解热；秋、冬季节天气干燥，服用蜂蜜可以滋阴润燥。

◎ 如何搭配药材、食材？

体内有留饮者，可合用甘遂半夏汤；心下坚满者，饮邪在上且肠燥，可合用半夏、白芍，消饮于上而降之。蜂蜜不仅能缓解甘遂、半夏等药物的峻烈之性，还能调和人体的气血，有助于消除体内的留饮，起到增效减毒等诸多作用。

在日常生活中，蜂蜜枸杞水有很好的降火功效，常可用来缓解口舌生疮，还能护眼明目，改善视力。蜂蜜红糖水可淡化色斑。雪梨蜂蜜水可止咳、醒酒。生姜蜂蜜水可缓解咽炎与痛经。

## 小验方

1. 治疗功能性便秘

蜂蜜50g，蜂王浆5g，调匀，直接口服，每日早、晚各1次温服。

2. 治疗产后血虚

蜂蜜50g，牛奶50ml，黑芝麻25g。黑芝麻捣碎，与牛奶、蜂蜜调和服用，早晨空腹温开水冲服。

3. 治疗小儿支气管哮喘

蜂蜜20g，鸡蛋2个。油煎鸡蛋，趁热加入蜂蜜，立刻食用，连服2~3个月。

# 十一、荷叶

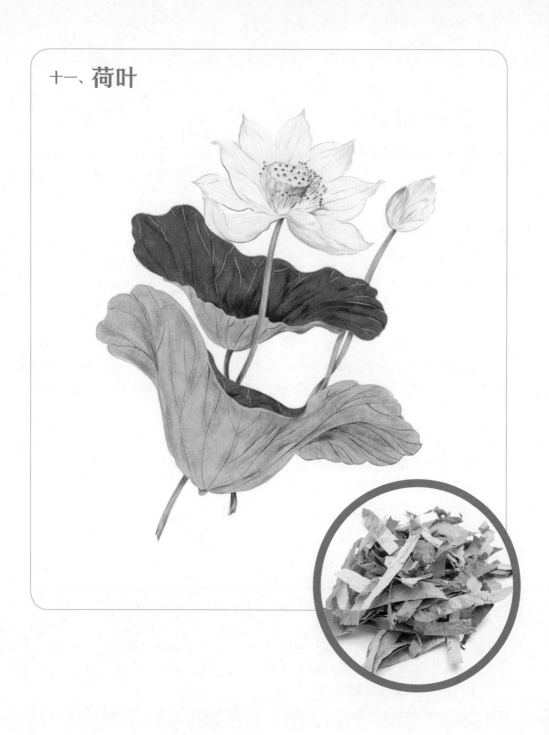

## 【广医药师谈选药】

◎ **哪里产的荷叶质量较好？**

中国是荷叶的优质产区，尤以杭州西湖产的荷叶质量为优。

◎ **如何辨别荷叶质量的好坏？**

以切片大、外观整洁、新鲜色绿、无虫蛀、干燥者为佳。

◎ **荷叶如何保存？**

荷叶饮片分为干荷叶和鲜荷叶。干荷叶可以在密封、干燥、避光、通风处保存。鲜荷叶可剪掉根部，冲洗，开水烫后沥干，放入保鲜袋，冷冻保存。

◎ **荷叶鲜用和干用有什么区别？**

鲜荷叶有消解脂肪、通便利尿的功效。干荷叶凉性更强一些，有清暑利湿、升阳止泻、祛瘀止血等功效。药用以干品为多，入饮食以鲜品更多。

## 【广医医师说功效】

◎ **药性与功效——清热解暑，升清止泻**

荷叶微苦，凉。归心、肝、胃、脾经。荷叶性凉，主要有清除暑热之邪的功效，也可治疗暑湿泄泻。另外，荷叶炒炭后收涩化瘀止血，用于多种出血症及产后血晕。荷叶出淤泥而不染，生于池塘，在水湿弥散之地可较好地生长，证明其有较好的化湿功效；荷叶生于夏日，炎炎夏日水上部分依旧能保持鲜绿，其除暑热的功效亦优。荷叶入脾、胃经，脾主升清，胃主降浊，具有调节脾胃之升清降浊功能。

◎ **适用人群——暑热来袭，湿邪泄泻，瘀血，出血者**

荷叶主要适用于暑热湿邪来袭，病发泄泻，体内瘀血过多或有出血症状的人群。

暑热来袭为主者，可见突发高热、头晕头痛、出汗、口干、口渴等。

湿邪泄泻为主者，可见头重如裹、腹泻、大便黏腻、四肢沉重等。

瘀血为主者，可见肌肤甲错、皮肤有瘀斑瘀点、面色晦暗、口唇青紫、身体有刺痛且痛处固定不移等。

出血为主者，可见消化道、呼吸道或皮肤部位出血，女性可见月经过多等。

◎ 适用病证

荷叶能清热、祛湿、解暑、止血、散瘀，可用于夏季感受暑热之邪、湿热泄泻，且可以降血糖，降血脂，保护免疫器官、增强免疫作用，抗癌，抗病毒等。还可用于头痛眩晕、身体浮肿、便血、崩漏、吐血、衄血、产后出血等病症。

◎ 什么样的人不适合用荷叶？

荷叶性味苦凉，气血虚弱体瘦者慎服。身体比较虚弱或脾胃虚寒严重的人群，尽量不要过多服用荷叶茶，容易引起身体不适、泄泻，甚至脱水。月经期的女性不要服用荷叶。荷叶畏桐油、茯苓，不可同用。

## 【 广医专家话食疗 】

◎ 荷叶食疗用法用量

荷叶性凉、苦，日常可用到 15g 左右。可以和粳米、冰糖一起煮荷叶粥，清热利湿、降血压、降血脂，也可以与绿茶一起冲泡水饮用，可排油减脂，瘦身减肥。

◎ 荷叶最适合什么季节服用？

荷叶一年四季皆可服用，但因其性凉，最适合夏季服用，能够清暑利湿降火，防止夏季中暑或湿气过多。

◎ 如何搭配药材、食材？

患有"三高"的人群，可以将荷叶与山楂搭配同用；与艾叶、侧柏叶、地黄同用，可治疗吐血衄血；与蒲黄、黄芩同用，治疗崩中下血。

在日常生活中，荷叶粥可以清凉解暑、降压降脂。搭配绿茶可以去油腻、减肥排毒。与白糖合用，可以治疗泄泻。与香油一起调匀可以治疗黄水疮。搭配冬瓜，可以清暑利尿，解除烦躁。

**小验方**

**1. 治疗高血压、高血脂**

鲜荷叶 2 张，山楂 50g，薏苡仁 50g。煮粥，加入适量冰糖，可作为早、晚餐。

**2. 治疗肥胖**

鲜荷叶 1 张，紫菜 20g。荷叶清水煮开，去渣取汁，倒入紫菜一起煮，餐前服用。

**3. 治疗皮肤出痱**

鲜荷叶 1 张，绿豆适量，煮水服用。

# 十二、黑芝麻

◎ 哪里产的黑芝麻好?

以河南省驻马店产的黑芝麻质量为佳。

◎ 如何辨别黑芝麻质量的好坏?

以颗粒完整、色黑鲜亮、无异味、断面色白、搓可掉色、味微香甜者
为佳。

◎ 黑芝麻如何保存?

黑芝麻可分为生熟两种,生芝麻可晒干后放入入塑料桶中,密封保存。
熟芝麻炒熟前应晒干,否则容易发霉,可密封后放入冰箱冷藏。

◎ 黑芝麻生用和熟用有什么区别?

黑芝麻可分为生用和熟用,生用可补肾阴、祛胃火,侧重于润肠通便。
熟制后更易被人体吸收,阴阳同补,且养胃。


【 广医医师说功效 】


◎ 药性与功效——滋补肝肾、益血润肠、通便

黑芝麻味甘,性平,归肝、肾、大肠经。其色黑,入肾经,可滋补肝
肾。黑芝麻为油性作物,含有大量的脂肪类物质,可润肠通便,治疗肠燥
津亏导致的便秘。

◎ 适用人群——肝肾不足、血虚、肠燥便秘

黑芝麻主要适用于肝肾阴精不足、血虚、肠燥便秘的人群,多用于平
素体质较差、血虚津亏、易腰膝酸软、大便干的人群。

肝肾阴精不足为主者,多见腰膝酸软、头晕、情绪抑郁、眼睛干涩,
男性可能出现阳强易举、遗精早泄等。

血虚为主者,可出现面色苍白、爪甲色淡、容易疲劳,女性可能出现

月经量少、月经后期等。

便秘为主者，多见解便难、大便干燥，可能会损伤肠络而出现少量出血症状等。

◎ 适用病证

黑芝麻可用于少白发、轻微贫血，黑芝麻的钙含量超过80％，可以补钙，且含有较多的钾，有利于排钠降压，保护心脏健康。

◎ 什么样的人不适合用黑芝麻？

因为黑芝麻富含维生素E，所以患有乳腺结节、乳腺增生、乳腺囊肿等乳腺疾病的人应尽量少吃黑芝麻。由于黑芝麻脂肪含量较高，为油性作物，可滑肠通便，所以经常腹泻或患有肠易激综合征的人应少吃黑芝麻。熟制的黑芝麻燥性过大，所以不适合内热上火之人服用。

【广医专家话食疗】

◎ 黑芝麻食疗用法用量

黑芝麻日常服用15~20g。可以与粳米、大枣一起煮粥，或与枸杞子一起研末服用。

◎ 黑芝麻最适合什么季节服用？

黑芝麻一年四季皆可服用，但是冬季服用效果最佳。黑芝麻色黑入肾，冬天阳气藏于肾中，此时服用黑芝麻顺四时节气及人体阴阳气血变化，对扶助人体正气，固护肾中真气具有较好的功效，所以冬季服用黑芝麻养肾最佳。

◎ 如何搭配药材、食材？

黑芝麻可搭配枸杞子、熟地黄同用，治疗头昏眼花、失眠健忘、腰膝酸软；配合何首乌、桑椹、枸杞子同用，治疗白发；炒熟研末同蜂蜜调服治疗产后便秘、习惯性便秘。

## 1. 治疗慢性腰痛

黑芝麻 30g，核桃仁 30g，洗净，泡入 500g 白酒中，密封半月。每日服用 2 次，每次 15g。

## 2. 治疗老年慢性气喘

黑芝麻 250g，白蜜 75g（蒸熟），生姜汁 5g，冰糖 75g（捣碎蒸）。将捣碎蒸好的冰糖溶于黑芝麻炒熟，凉后倒入生姜汁拌好，再炒后，放凉。拌上蒸熟的白蜜，放入瓶中，早晚各一勺。

## 3. 治疗妊娠便秘

黑芝麻 60g，杏仁 5g，核桃仁 10g。捣碎，加水蒸熟，加入红糖调和。隔日服 1 次，每日 3 次。

## 4. 治疗老年性便秘

黑芝麻 15g，粳米 150g，蜂蜜适量。将黑芝麻炒熟，粳米加水煮熟后倒入黑芝麻，一起煮烂后稍放凉，加入适量蜂蜜拌匀。每日 2 次，早晚各 1 次服用。

# 十三、马齿苋

## 【广医药师谈选药】

◎ 马齿苋入药用哪部分？

马齿苋科植物马齿苋的干燥地上部分。

◎ 如何辨别马齿苋质量的好坏？

以株小、叶多、质嫩、色青绿者为佳。

◎ 马齿苋如何保存？

马齿苋可分为鲜品和干品，新鲜的马齿苋可用保鲜膜包好放入冰箱冷藏，也可用盐开水烫熟捞出沥干水分，晒干放进干净的塑料袋，放在阴凉处储存。干燥的马齿苋要注意防潮，放在阴凉干燥处保存，避免阳光照晒。

◎ 马齿苋入药宜怎样用？

马齿苋宜用鲜品，可清热解毒，凉血止血，止痢。

## 【广医医师说功效】

◎ **药性与功效——清热解毒，凉血止血，止痢**

马齿苋味微酸，性寒，气微，归肝、大肠经。本品性寒，味微酸，可清热解毒，凉血止血。酸主收涩，可治疗热毒血痢、泄泻。入肝经，有清热凉血、收敛止血的功效，可治疗大肠湿热下注。外用可治疗痈肿疔疮、丹毒、蛇虫咬伤、湿疹。

◎ **适用人群——湿热下注、热毒血痢、皮肤出疹**

马齿苋主要用于体内热毒炽盛、湿热下注的人群，多用于痢疾、里急后重、便血崩漏者。

湿热下注为主者，多见腹痛泄泻、里急后重、白带发黄、小便短赤、湿热淋证等。

热毒血痢为主者，多见高热神昏、黏液脓血便、腹痛、肛门灼热、里急后重等。

皮肤出疹为主者，多见皮肤湿疹、湿疮、流黄脓等。

◎ 适用病证

马齿苋具有清热解毒的疗效，可用于治疗痢疾、便血，还能利尿祛湿，治疗各类湿疹、湿疮。此外，还能降脂，具有改善高脂血症的疗效。

◎ 什么样的人不适合用马齿苋？

马齿苋性寒，脾胃虚寒者忌服；肠滑泄泻者也属于中焦阳气不足，无法固摄，故也应忌服。且马齿苋性寒滑利，孕妇应慎用。

【 广医专家话食疗 】

◎ 马齿苋食疗用法用量

马齿苋性寒，一般不可以多食。日常生活中，干马齿苋用 12~16g，新鲜马齿苋用 35~65g 为佳。凉拌马齿苋可以用 250~300g，煮粥时用 300g 左右，炒鸡蛋时用 80g 左右。

◎ 马齿苋最适合什么季节服用？

马齿苋性寒、微酸，多在 3—8 月服用。

◎ 如何搭配药材、食材？

马齿苋性寒、微酸，与黄芩、黄连搭配，可以治疗里急后重；与地榆、槐角、凤尾草同用，可治疗大肠湿热、便血、痔疮出血；搭配茜草、苎麻根、侧柏叶，可治疗血热妄行、崩漏下血，也可单味药捣汁服用。

在日常生活中，马齿苋可与芡实、瘦肉同煮，清热解毒，祛湿止带；搭配白糖、食醋，发挥驱虫的功效；搭配鸡蛋一起炒，清热解毒，止痢疾，益气补虚，用于湿热久痢；和粳米一起煮粥，治疗痢疾便血、湿热腹泻；搭配鲜藕绞汁，可以清热止血。

### 1. 治疗湿热或热毒痢疾、泄泻

马齿苋 30g（鲜者加倍），大米 100g，白糖适量。煮粥，每日 1 剂，连服 5 日。

### 2. 治疗大肠病变引起的便血

鲜马齿苋 100g，槐花 30g，粳米 100g，红糖 20g。煮粥，槐花后入，每日早晚两次分服。

### 3. 治疗赤白带下

马齿苋 250g，鸡蛋 2 个，马齿苋捣烂绞汁，与鸡蛋清搅匀，沸水冲服。每日服用 2 次。

### 4. 治疗小儿钩虫病

马齿苋 200~250g，食醋 30g，白糖适量。马齿苋煎浓汁，去渣，加入食醋、白糖调匀。1 次或 2 次空腹温热饮用，连服 3 天。如需再服，隔半月。

# 十四、蒲公英

## 【广医药师谈选药】

◎ 蒲公英的入药部位是哪里？

　　菊科植物蒲公英、碱地蒲公英或同属数种植物的干燥全草。

◎ 哪里产的蒲公英质量好？

　　以河北、四川等地产的蒲公英质量为佳。

◎ 如何辨别蒲公英质量的好坏？

　　以叶多、色灰绿、带根者为佳。

◎ 蒲公英如何保存？

　　将新鲜的蒲公英洗净后放在干燥通风处自然风干，或沥干后套上保鲜膜放入冰箱冷冻，食用时再解冻。干品蒲公英可直接放在阴凉通风处，避光保存。

◎ 蒲公英的根、叶功效有什么区别？

　　蒲公英全身皆可入药，根部侧重于肝脏的解毒清火，叶侧重于消炎解毒，用于牙龈上火或者口腔溃疡等症状。

## 【广医医师说功效】

◎ 药性与功效——清热解毒、消肿散结、利湿通淋

　　蒲公英性寒，味苦、甘，归肝、胃经。其性寒，可清热解毒，用于痈肿疗疮、乳痈、肺痈、肠痈、瘰疬；可以清肝明目，消肿散结，治疗肝火上炎引起的目赤肿痛。其味苦，能降能燥，治疗湿热黄疸、热淋涩痛。此外，本品可单用取汁点眼，也可外敷治疗痈肿疗疮。

◎ 适用人群——内外热毒疮痈诸证、湿热黄疸、淋证

　　蒲公英性寒，以味苦为主，主要用于内外热毒炽盛，湿热下注诸证。多用于平素体热、易上火的人群。

内外热毒诸证，多见痈肿疔疮、乳痈、肺痈吐脓、咽喉肿痛、毒蛇咬伤等。

湿热黄疸，多见发热、目黄、身黄、小便黄。

淋证，多见小便短赤涩痛、淋沥不尽等。

◎ 适用病证

蒲公英具有清热解毒的功效，可用于治疗感冒引起的咽喉肿痛，还可用于治疗慢性胃炎、肠炎、黄疸等。

◎ 什么样的人不适合用蒲公英？

蒲公英性寒，凡是脾胃虚寒、阳虚体质的人群，宫寒的女性，有阴寒类病证者，皆不适合食用蒲公英。应用蒲公英时，用量过大会引发胃脘疼痛等症状，严重者甚至发生缓泻，临床应用应引起注意。

## 【广医专家话食疗】

◎ **蒲公英食疗用法用量**

新鲜的蒲公英成人每天用量不宜超过 60g，小儿减半；干蒲公英成人每天用量不宜超过 12g，小儿减半。蒲公英食用方法较多，可生炒、凉拌、煮粥或做馅。

◎ **蒲公英最适合什么季节服用？**

蒲公英性寒，夏、秋季节比较热的时候服用最好。春天也可服用蒲公英，有利于提高免疫力。

◎ **如何搭配药材、食材？**

蒲公英可与瓜蒌、金银花同用，治疗乳痈肿痛；与金银花、野菊花、紫花地丁同用，治疗痈肿疔疮；搭配大黄、牡丹皮、桃仁，治疗肠痈腹痛；与鱼腥草、冬瓜仁、芦根等同用，治疗肺痈吐脓；搭配夏枯草、连翘、浙贝母，治疗瘰疬；配伍板蓝根、玄参，治疗咽喉肿痛。

在日常食疗时，炒菜可搭配猪肉、牛肉等，起到清热解毒、养阴护阳的功效；搭配玉米芯代茶饮，治疗热淋、小便短赤；和鸡蛋一起煎，可以缓解风热导致的烦躁不安、胎动不安、咽喉肿痛等。

1. 治疗热毒炽盛、内外疖肿

   鲜蒲公英 35g，粳米 150g，煮粥，餐时服用。

2. 治疗咳痰黄稠

   鲜蒲公英 60g，猪肉 200g，煮熟后食用。每日 1 次。

3. 治疗脚气

   鲜蒲公英 15~35g，煮开，晾温泡脚，每日 2 次，一次 15~30 分钟。也可鲜品捣烂外敷，杀菌，治脚气。

# 十五、莲子

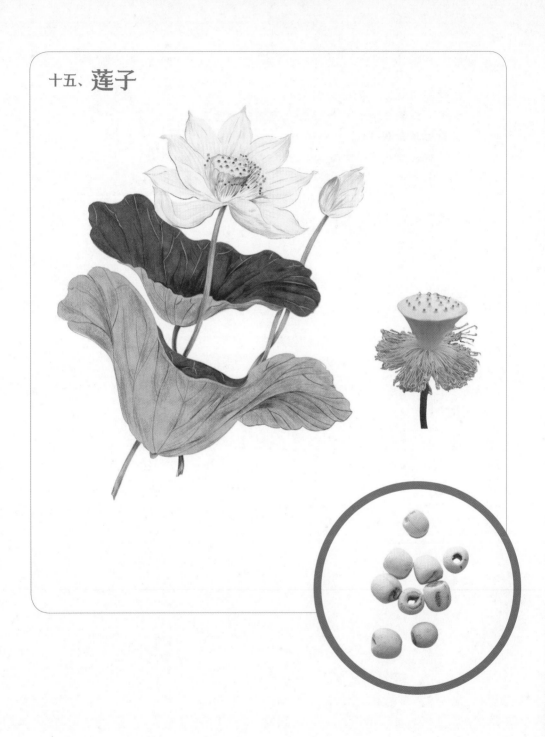

## 【广医药师谈选药】

◎ 莲子入药用用哪部分?

莲子为睡莲科植物莲的干燥成熟种子，去心生用。

◎ 哪里产的莲子好?

莲子以福建省建宁县产的建莲，浙江省武义县宣平产的宣莲，江西省广昌县产的白莲、湖南省湘潭市产的湘莲质量较好。

◎ 如何辨别莲子质量的好坏?

以个大、饱满、表面整齐、无杂质、无异味、颜色淡黄、有光泽者为佳。

◎ 莲子如何保存?

将成熟的莲子摘出，保留绿色外壳，放入冰箱冷藏储存。也可以晒干后放入密闭的容器或塑料袋中储存。

## 【广医医师说功效】

◎ 药性与功效——补脾止泻、止带、益肾涩精、养心安神

莲子甘、涩，性平。归脾、肾、心经。本品甘、平，入心、肾经，能养心、益肾、安神，交通心肾，治疗心悸失眠。本品归脾经，可补脾止泻，治疗脾虚泄泻。可固涩止带，治疗女性带下病症。味甘而涩，故能涩精止遗。

◎ 适用人群——脾虚泄泻、脾肾亏虚、心肾不交

莲子主要适用于脾肾亏虚、心肾不交的人群，多用于平素脾虚泄泻、虚烦、心悸、失眠，女子带下，男子遗精者。此外，莲子属于药食两用的中药，无疾病的人群在平日适当服用莲子，有较好的保健效果。

脾虚泄泻为主者，多见四肢乏力、泄泻、面色萎黄等。

脾肾亏虚为主者，多见腰膝酸软，女子带下清稀，男子遗精、滑精等。

心肾不交为主者，多见虚烦、心悸、失眠、眩晕、健忘、耳鸣等。

◎ 适用病证

莲子具有补益脾肾的功效，可用于治疗脾肾亏虚导致的腹泻、乏力，同时还能养心安神，治疗心悸、失眠。

◎ 什么样的人不适合用莲子？

因为莲子味甘而涩，收敛固涩作用较强，因此肠燥津亏引起的大便燥结者不宜食用莲子。

## 【广医专家话食疗】

◎ 莲子食疗用法用量

日常每天服用控制在 15~30g。可以熬粥、煲汤、做羹。

◎ 莲子最适合什么季节服用？

莲子药性平和，不必拘于四时变化，一年四季皆可服用。

◎ 如何搭配药材、食材？

莲子搭配人参、茯苓、白术，治疗脾虚久泻、食欲不振；搭配山药、白术、茯苓，治疗脾虚带下；搭配山药、芡实、山茱萸，治疗脾肾亏虚、带下清稀、腰膝酸软；与龙骨、芡实同用，治疗遗精、滑精；搭配酸枣仁、茯神、远志，治疗心悸失眠。

在日常生活中，可以和银耳、冰糖一起做羹，滋阴润肺、养胃生津；和百合、枸杞子一起煲汤清心去热；和百合、瘦肉一起熬粥，补脾肺、益气。

1. **治疗心悸怔忡、虚烦失眠**

   莲子15g，红糖10g，糯米150g。去莲心，熬粥，每日1次，餐时服用。

2. **治疗中老年人脾肺气虚咳嗽**

   莲子25g，百合25g，猪瘦肉300g，各种调料适量，煮烂。分数次服用，每周2次。

3. **治疗女子带下**

   莲子15g，白果20g，乌骨鸡1只（约600g）。将莲子、白果放入处理好的鸡腹中，加入调料、清水炖烂，每日1次。

4. **治疗贫血**

   莲子25g，龙眼肉15g，糯米50g，同煮熬粥，温热服用，每日2次。

5. **治疗血虚头晕**

   莲子30g，大枣15枚，龙眼肉20g，花生米20g。加水煮烂食用，每日2次。

# 十六、姜（生姜、干姜）

第二章　常用中药使用指导

◎ 姜的外皮能不能入药？

中药里的姜是以姜科植物姜的根茎入药，连皮使用。姜的外皮也可单独入药。

◎ 哪里产的姜好？

全国大部地区有产，以四川、山东产的姜最为有名。干姜尤以四川产者为佳。

◎ 如何辨别姜质量的好坏？

生姜以块大、丰满、质嫩者为佳。干姜以色白、粉性足、味辣者为佳。

◎ 姜如何保存？

生姜宜置阴凉潮湿处，或埋入湿沙内，防冻；干姜干燥阴凉处保存即可。

◎ 生姜和干姜有什么区别？

姜饮片主要是指生姜和干姜，前者解表散寒效果好，后者温中散寒效果好。而生姜皮利水消肿的功效较强。

【 广医医师说功效 】

◎ 药性与功效——温肺、散寒

生姜味辛，性温，归肺、脾、胃经，故能解表散寒、温肺止咳，同时还有温中止呕的作用；而干姜性更热，有良好的温中散寒、回阳通脉作用。此外，生姜还兼有一定的解毒作用，解鱼蟹等食物中毒，又可用于炮制半夏、天南星，以减除它们的毒性。

◎ 适用人群——阳虚体质，脾胃虚寒

姜一般人群均可食用。尤其适用于脾胃阳虚、体质较弱的人群，多用于平素怕冷、容易感冒者，以及肠胃虚寒者。

外感风寒为主者，多见恶寒、鼻塞、流清涕、头痛身痛或有咳嗽等。

脾胃虚寒为主者，多见胃脘隐隐作痛、呕吐、腹痛腹泻、纳食不香等。

◎ 适用病证

姜可用于关节炎、牙痛、重症呕吐、急性胃肠炎、胃及十二指肠溃疡、急性肠梗阻、蛔虫病、小儿腹泻、急性细菌性痢疾、疟疾、褥疮等疾病见上述证候者，以及中毒急救、晕车的治疗。

◎ 什么样的人不适合用姜？

因为姜性质偏温热，因此阴虚内热及邪热亢盛者不宜使用。同时因为其味辛刺激，所以孕妇应当慎用。

【广医专家话食疗】

◎ 姜食疗用法用量

食疗用生姜可与茶同饮，用去皮生姜 5~10g。居家佐餐如炒菜、煲汤、煮粥等，鲜姜可以用 30~60g，干姜多与其他调味品同用，用 3~10g。一次服用姜不宜过多。

◎ 姜最适合什么季节服用？

姜日常皆可食用，但秋天不宜多用。秋天多燥，燥气伤肺，如食生姜，辛温发散，易泻肺气，故不宜多服。

◎ 如何搭配药材、食材？

姜辛散温通，但作用较弱，用于风寒感冒时配桂枝、羌活等辛温解表药。治痰多咳嗽，恶寒头痛者，每与麻黄、苦杏仁同用。治脾胃寒证，宜与高良姜、胡椒、党参、白术等温里、补气药同用。对胃寒呕吐最为适合，可配伍高良姜、豆蔻等温胃止呕药。

在日常炒菜时可以搭配凉性食物，如苦瓜、荸荠、百合、柚子、梨等，姜性属温热，可防止体内寒气加重。也可与热性食物如羊肉同用，羊肉补血温阳、生姜止痛、祛风湿，祛腥膻味，以增强温阳祛寒的功效。

◎ 生姜、干姜食疗时如何选择？

生姜与干姜都是姜的块茎，都具有散寒温肺的食疗功效。生姜发散力比较强，有发汗的作用，所以有外感时更适用，醒脾开胃的作用好。而干姜更为辛热，可温中逐寒、回阳通脉，治心腹冷痛、吐泻、四肢发冷、妇女痛经等疗效更好。

## 小验方

1. 治疗风寒感冒、咳嗽

   茶叶10g，生姜10g（去皮切片），同煎水，饭后服。

2. 治疗寒性痛经

   干姜、大枣、红糖各30g。干姜洗净切片，大枣洗净去核，与红糖共煎汤服；或生姜20g切丝，红糖适量，沸水冲开后加盖3分钟，趁热代茶饮。

3. 治疗胃寒呕吐

   生姜榨汁，加入热水和蜂蜜调味饮用。

# 十七、大枣

## 【广医药师谈选药】

◎ 大枣的药用部位是什么？

大枣以鼠李科植物枣的成熟果实入药。

◎ 哪里产的大枣好？

山东、河南产的大枣质量较优。

◎ 如何辨别大枣质量的好坏？

大枣以果实粒大均匀、肉质厚、色光泽、味甜者为佳。酸枣仁以种子颗粒饱满、表面平滑有光泽、色黑褐者为佳。

◎ 大枣如何保存？

新鲜大枣适宜晒干后保存，置于干燥阴凉处即可。

## 【广医医师说功效】

◎ 药性与功效——补益、安神

大枣味道甘甜，性温，具有补益作用，尤擅于养血安神。

◎ 适用人群——平和质、阴虚体质

大枣适用于普通人平时养生服用，对脾虚、血虚、妇人脏躁、失眠、阴虚盗汗尤为适宜。

脾虚证为主者，多见饮食不佳、消瘦、倦怠乏力、便溏等。

血虚为主者，多见面色苍白、唇色爪甲淡白无华、头发枯焦、头晕目眩、肢体麻木、心悸怔忡等。

脏躁、失眠为主者，多见精神恍惚、哭笑无常、情绪波动较大、心烦失眠、健忘等。

◎ 适用病证

大枣可用于日常服用以提高免疫力，保肝护肝，预防心血管疾病、贫血。对于已经发生的心血管疾病、贫血、失眠、情志抑郁等见上述证候者也有很好的疗效。

◎ 什么样的人不适合用大枣？

因为大枣为补益之品，因此湿热、痰湿体质者不适合服用。

【广医专家话食疗】

◎ 大枣食疗用法用量

大枣药性甘润和缓，大枣用于日常熬粥、煲汤，可根据需要调整用量，一般用 30~100g，代茶饮用 10~15g。

◎ 大枣最适合什么季节服用？

大枣四季皆可服用，因为其具有滋补的作用，所以尤其适合冬季养生。

◎ 如何搭配药材、食材？

大枣药性平和，可与多种药材搭配。取其补中益气疗效时，尤其是气虚较明显时常常佐入白术、人参等；治疗脏躁等，常与小麦、甘草合用；治疗失眠时常与黄芪、当归、远志、生地黄、龙眼肉等药材选择配伍。此外，大枣与部分药性峻烈或有毒的药物同用，还有保护胃气，缓和其毒烈药性之效。

在日常炒菜时常与百合、茯苓、当归、龙眼肉等食材搭配，以增强补益、养血、安神的效用。

小验方

1. 日常养生及补血

大枣 100g 洗净放入锅内煮沸，然后改用文火煮 15~20 分钟，取水饮用。

2. 治疗贫血

大枣 50g，姜 5g，赤砂糖 10g。大枣与生姜一同放入砂锅内，加适量清水，文火煮半分钟，加入红糖搅匀即成。

# 第二节
## 用于保健食品的中药

## 一、黄芪

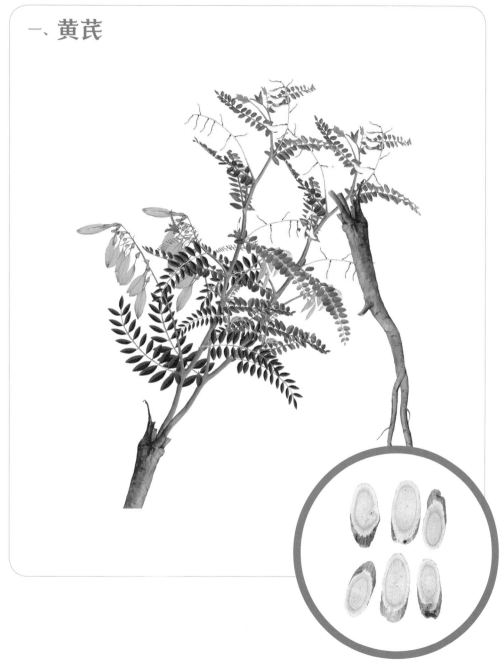

◎ 黄芪的药用部位是什么？

　　以豆科植物蒙古黄芪或膜荚黄芪的根入药。

◎ 哪里产的黄芪好？

　　内蒙古、山西、黑龙江等地产的黄芪质量最优。

◎ 如何辨别黄芪质量的好坏？

　　以根部粗壮，皱纹少、质坚而绵，粉性足，味甜者为佳。

◎ 黄芪如何保存？

　　黄芪饮片置于干燥阴凉处即可。

◎ 黄芪生用和蜜炙用有什么区别？

　　黄芪饮片分为生黄芪和蜜炙黄芪，前者益气固表效果好，后者健脾补中效果好。

【 广医医师说功效 】

◎ 药性与功效——健脾补中、升阳举陷、益卫固表、利尿、托毒生肌

　　黄芪性温味甘，归脾、肺经，具有良好的健脾益肺功效。此外，本品还兼有一定的补气行血功效，与活血药物同用可以治疗痹证及中风后遗症。

◎ 适用人群——脾气虚弱、肺虚自汗、疮疡难溃

　　黄芪主要适用于脾肺气虚的人群，多用于体形偏瘦、平素气短、少语懒言、咳喘自汗、神疲乏力、浮肿尿少者。

　　脾气虚弱为主者，多见倦怠乏力、食少便溏、消化不良、腹痛腹泻等。

　　肺气虚弱为主者，多见咳喘日久、气短、神志恍惚、乏力、自汗、小便多等。

气血亏虚为主者，多见面色苍白、少气懒言、饮食减少、自汗乏力、疮疡难溃、溃疡难收等。

◎ 适用病证

黄芪可用于过敏性鼻炎、慢性鼻炎、上呼吸道感染、心绞痛、骨质疏松、关节炎、慢性肾炎、慢性肝炎、小儿哮喘、冠心病、产后非感染性发热等疾病属脾气虚弱、肺气虚弱、气血亏虚证候的治疗。

◎ 什么样的人不适合用黄芪？

因为黄芪性质甘温，而且有补气升阳作用，因此外感风热咳嗽、平素怕热喜凉、胃热喜饮冷水、大便秘结者不适合服用黄芪。

若服用黄芪后出现怕热、咽干、便秘者应该停用，可适当服用黄连水缓解症状。


【 广医专家话食疗 】


◎ 黄芪食疗用法用量

黄芪甘甜微温，日常代茶饮可以用 5~15g。居家佐餐如炒菜、煲汤、煮粥等，可以用 10~30g。

◎ 黄芪最适合什么季节服用？

黄芪四季皆可服用，因为其具有补气升阳的作用，所以尤其适合于秋、冬季节服用。

◎ 如何搭配药材、食材？

黄芪甘甜微温，取其健脾补中时，常配合人参或白术等增强其健脾补中的功效；治疗肺气虚弱、咳喘日久、气短神疲、自汗等，常与紫菀、款冬花、苦杏仁等合用。

常与当归、白术、茯苓等搭配，起到健脾补气的功效；煮粥时常可搭配薏苡仁、山药等健脾补气；煲汤时常可搭配党参、苦杏仁、防风等补肺益气。

◎ 黄芪、人参食疗时如何选择?

黄芪与人参都是甘温之品,都具有补气生津、生血的食疗功效,常搭配使用,可互相提高疗效。与人参相比,黄芪还能利水消肿,因此如有脾肺虚弱、浮肿尿少选用黄芪更为适宜。

小验方

1. 治疗慢性鼻炎

黄芪 15g,白术 12g,防风 10g。煲汤,每日早、晚各 1 次温服。

2. 治疗骨质疏松

黄芪 30g,桂枝 10g,白芍 15g,生姜 3 片,大枣 12 枚。煲汤,每日早、晚各 1 次温服。

## 二、当归

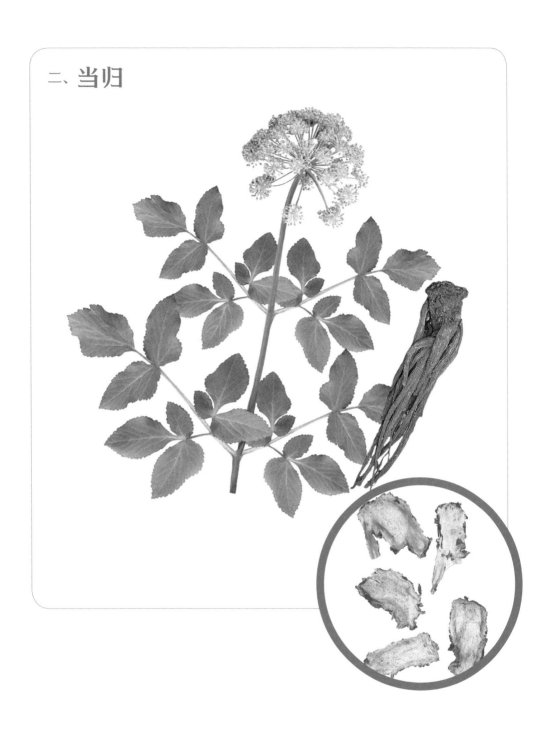

◎ 当归入药用哪个部分？

以伞形科植物当归的根入药。

◎ 哪里产的当归好？

以甘肃省东南部的岷县的产量大，质量好。其次，陕西、四川、云南、湖北等地也有栽培。

◎ 如何辨别当归质量的好坏？

以主根粗长、油润、肉质饱满、断面色黄白、气浓香者为佳。

◎ 当归如何保存？

当归饮片置于干燥阴凉处即可。

◎ 当归生用和酒制用有什么区别？

当归饮片分为生当归和酒制当归，前者补血养血效果好，后者活血补血效果好。

【 广医医师说功效 】

◎ 药性与功效——补血调经、活血止痛、润肠通便

当归味甘、辛，性温，归肝、心、脾经，具有补益作用，能补血调经，治疗血虚引起的月经量少；其药性辛温，能活血止痛，治疗血瘀引起的疼痛。此外，本品还兼有一定的润肠通便作用，可以治疗肠燥便秘。

◎ 适用人群——阴虚体质，咽干久咳、虚烦失眠

当归主要适用于肝、心、脾经血虚的人群，多用于体形偏瘦、心慌气短、容易自汗、血虚痛经、大便偏干、小便量多清长者。

气血两虚为主者，多见心慌气短、乏力、自汗、失眠、健忘、懒言等。

血虚血瘀为主者，多见失眠、痛经、口渴喜温水、神志恍惚、舌质偏暗等。

虚寒腹痛为主者，多见怕冷、乏力、腹痛、饮食减少、大便偏稀等。

◎ 适用病证

当归可用于缺血性中风、血栓闭塞性脉管炎、高血压、缺铁性贫血、痛经、慢性腹泻等疾病见气血两虚、血虚血瘀、虚寒腹痛证候者的治疗。

◎ 什么样的人不适合用当归？

因为当归性质略偏辛温，而且有和血补血作用，因此肝胆火旺，平素怕热喜凉、胃热喜饮凉水者不适合服用当归。

若服用当归后出现怕热、胃热、腹泻者应该停用，可适当服用黄连水缓解症状。


【 广医专家话食疗 】


◎ 当归食疗用法用量

当归药性甘温和缓，日常代茶饮可以用 5~15g。居家佐餐如炒菜、煲汤、煮粥等，饮片可以用 10~30g。

◎ 当归最适合什么季节服用？

当归四季皆可服用，因为其具有补血活血的作用，所以尤其适合于秋、冬季节服用。

◎ 如何搭配药材、食材？

当归辛温甘甜，取其补血养虚功效时，尤其是滋补心脾气血时常常佐入红糖或蜂蜜等增强其补血养虚的功效；治疗血瘀经闭者，腹痛喜温喜按、手脚心寒冷等，常与桃仁、红花、阿胶、艾叶等合用。

当归常与黄芪、肉桂、生姜等搭配，起到温阳补血的功效；煮粥时常可搭配桃仁、红花等消肿止痛；煲汤时常可搭配人参、黄芪、肉桂等补气养血。

◎ 当归、黄芪食疗时如何选择?

　　当归与黄芪都是甘温之品,都具有补血养虚的食疗功效,常搭配使用,可互相提高疗效。与黄芪相比,当归还能润肠通便,因此如有血虚肠燥、大便燥结者选用当归更为适宜。

> **小验方**
>
> **治疗失血后气血耗伤,或气虚血亏、体倦乏力、头昏**
>
> 　　当归10g,黄芪60g,煎水饮。每次饮用100ml,每日2次。

# 三、车前子

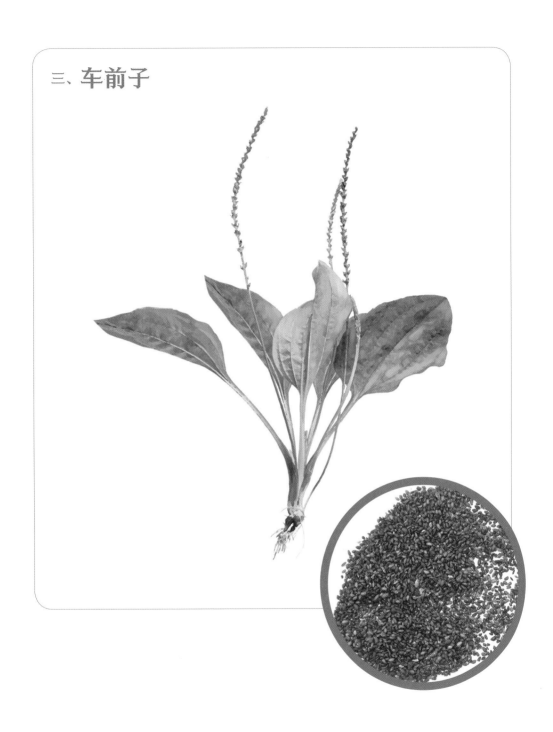

◎ 车前子有大有小，哪种更好？

大粒的车前子主要产于南方各地，而小粒的则主要产于华北、东北、西北等地，两者只是品种不同，从质量上来说没有明显的差别。

◎ 如何辨别车前子质量的好坏？

以粒大、均匀饱满、色棕红者为佳。

◎ 车前子如何保存？

车前子晒干后通常可以保存很长时间（1年左右），放在密封罐中置于阴凉干燥处即可。

◎ 车前子生用、炒用和盐水炒用有什么区别？

车前子饮片分为生车前子、炒车前子和盐水炒车前子。生用有利水作用，尤其是利尿效果好；炒后寒性减弱，祛湿止泻效果好；盐炒则主要用于补肝肾、明目。

【广医医师说功效】

◎ 药性与功效——清热、利尿、止泻、明目、祛痰

车前子味甘淡，中医认为淡味的中药具有利水渗湿的功效，其药性微偏寒，因此能够清热利水；车前子可以入肺、肝、肾、膀胱经而清除这些脏腑的湿热，因此该药还有清热止泻、清肺祛痰、清肝明目的功效。

◎ 适用人群——湿热体质，小便不畅、腹泻下利、眼睛干涩

车前子主要适用于湿热体质的人群，尤其是肺、肝、肾、膀胱内有湿热蕴结的患者。多用于平素怕热、眼睛干涩红肿、咳喘甚至咯鲜血、腹部胀满、肢体浮肿、小便不畅、大便溏薄、妇女黄白带偏多者。

肺热咳喘为主者，多见咳喘、咳吐黄痰、胸痛，甚至咯血，咽干，烦热等。

肝火目赤为主者，多见心烦易怒、口苦咽干、眼睛干涩或红肿疼痛、眼屎多、小便黄等。

湿热泻痢为主者，多见腹部胀满、食后胸膈不适、腹泻下利、肠鸣腹痛等。

湿热小便不利为主者，多见肢体浮肿，小便滞涩或淋沥不畅，或尿热尿痛，甚至尿血，妇女黄白带偏多。

◎ 适用病证

车前子可用于哮喘、肺炎、腹泻、胃肠功能紊乱、急性肾小球肾炎、慢性肾炎、结膜炎、视疲劳等疾病见湿热内蕴证候者的治疗。

◎ 什么样的人不适合用车前子？

因为车前子性质略偏寒凉，因此体质虚弱，过度劳累，平素怕冷喜暖、阳气不足，肾虚滑精者慎服。中医认为"诸子皆降"，车前子药性渗利向下，平时有胃下垂、子宫脱垂、脱肛等疾病的人群也不适宜服用。

若服用车前子后出现怕冷、胃寒、遗精滑泄者应该停用，可适当服用桂皮等缓解症状。

【广医专家话食疗】

◎ 车前子食疗用法用量

车前子药性甘淡和缓，日常代茶饮可以用 5~10g。居家佐餐如煲汤、煮粥等，可以用 10~15g。

◎ 车前子最适合什么季节服用？

车前子四季皆可服用。因为其具有清热、利尿、明目的作用，尤其适合于夏、秋季节服用。

◎ 如何搭配药材、食材？

车前子甘淡微寒，取其清热利水，治疗血热尿血时，常常搭配栀子、小蓟、白茅根等；对于老年前列腺增生或前列腺炎，小便淋沥不畅者，常与生地黄、冬葵子、石韦等合用；用于治疗眼睛干涩或肿胀不适，常配合决明子、菊花、枸杞子等增强清肝明目效果。

煮粥时常可搭配薏苡仁、白扁豆、山药等清热健脾止泻；煲汤时常可搭配乌鸡、鸭肉、鲤鱼等清热利水消肿。

◎ 车前子、车前草食疗时如何选择？

车前子与车前草功用相似，都具有清热、利尿、止泻等食疗功效，但车前草还有清热解毒的功效，内服可治疗热毒疮疖、血热尿血、湿热腹泻等；也常用鲜车前草叶捣碎外敷伤口，有止血、消炎、促进愈合的效果。

### 小验方

1. 治疗妇女白带过多

车前根 9g，捣烂，用糯米淘米水兑服。

2. 治疗高血压

车前子、鱼腥草各 30g，水煎服。

## 四、三七

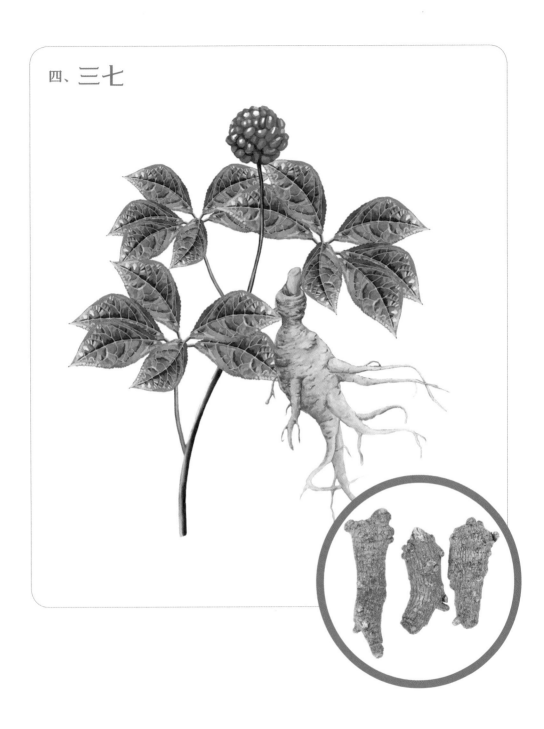

◎ 三七的药用部位有哪些?

三七为五加科多年生草本植物,临床中以根、根茎作为三七饮片入药。

◎ 如何辨别三七质量的好坏?

三七以身干、个大、体重、质坚、表皮光滑、断面灰绿色或灰黑色者为佳。

◎ 三七如何保存?

三七干品受潮后易发霉,所以应将干品用厚皮纸或布袋包好,置于阴凉通风处。

【 广医医师说功效 】

◎ **药性与功效——化瘀止血,活血定痛**

三七味甘、微苦,性温,功擅止血,又能活血化瘀,对人体内外各种出血,无论有无瘀滞,均可应用,尤以有瘀滞者为宜。此外,本品可活血化瘀而消肿止痛,为治瘀血诸证之佳品,伤科之要药。凡跌打损伤,或筋骨折伤,瘀血肿痛等,本品皆为首选药物。

◎ **适用人群——血瘀体质,跌打损伤、心胃疼痛、虚损劳伤**

三七主要适合以下症状属瘀血阻滞者:吐血、衄血、咯血、尿血、便血等人体内外各种出血;大肠下血、妇人血崩、产后出血多等下部出血;跌打损伤、筋断骨折、瘀血肿痛;痈疽疮疡、心胃疼痛。此外,三七尚有补虚强壮作用,适合虚损劳伤之人。

◎ **适用病证**

三七可用于跌打损伤、痛经、高血压、肝炎、心胃疼痛等疾病见瘀血内阻证候者的治疗。

◎ 什么样的人不适合用三七?

因三七具有活血化瘀的作用,故孕妇忌用。因气血亏虚所致的痛经、月经失调,表现为经期或经后小腹隐痛喜按的妇女忌用。

【广医专家话食疗】

◎ 三七食疗用法用量

三七的食用方法有两种:三七可以粉碎成三七粉,直接用开水冲服,每日2次,每次3~5g。三七还可以炖鸡或炖排骨,用量为15g左右,有益气养血,滋养强壮的作用,治疗崩漏、产后虚弱、自汗、盗汗等,以及老年人头痛、腰肌酸软无力等症。

◎ 三七最适合什么季节服用?

一年四季皆可服用。

◎ 如何搭配药材、食材?

若治咯血、吐血、衄血、尿血、便血,三七可单用,也可与花蕊石、血余炭合用。三七同鸡炖食,主要取其补益气血功效,用于气血不足而有瘀滞者,也可用于冠心病、脑血管病及跌打损伤等。

小验方

1. 治疗吐血、衄血
   三七粉5g,米汤送服。
2. 治疗血淋
   三七粉5g,灯心草、姜汤送服。

五、麦冬

◎ 麦冬入药用哪部分?

以百合科植物麦冬的块根入药。

◎ 哪里产的麦冬好?

浙江产的麦冬质量较优。

◎ 如何辨别麦冬质量的好坏?

以表面淡黄白色、身干、个肥大、质软、半透明、有香气、嚼之发黏者为佳。

◎ 麦冬如何保存?

麦冬含有较多糖类成分,易吸潮泛油,若需长时间保存,应放置在密闭容器中,冷藏避光保存。置阴凉干燥处,防潮。

【广医医师说功效】

◎ 药性与功效——养阴、润肺、益胃、清心

麦冬味甘、性微寒,具有补益作用,入肺、胃经,故能养阴润肺、益胃生津;其味微苦,又入心经,中医认为苦味中药能够清热泻火,故能清心除烦,有良好的清心安神作用。

◎ 适用人群——阴虚体质,咽干久咳、虚烦失眠

麦冬主要适用于肺、胃、心阴虚内热的人群,多用于体形偏瘦、平素怕热、容易盗汗、失眠、口渴喜饮凉水、大便偏干、小便量少偏黄者。

阴虚肺燥为主者,多见干咳少痰、咳血、咽干、嘶哑、烦热、盗汗等。

阴虚胃热为主者,多见口干唇燥、嘈杂、干呕、饮食减少、食后胸膈不适、大便干结等。

虚热扰心为主者,多见失眠、心悸、神志恍惚、情绪不能自主、口苦、

小便黄等。

◎ 适用病证

麦冬可用于肺结核、肺炎、咽喉炎、充血性心力衰竭、慢性肺源性心脏病、冠状动脉粥样硬化性心脏病、病毒性心肌炎、慢性萎缩性胃炎、糖尿病等疾病见阴虚肺燥、阴虚胃热、虚热扰心证候者的治疗。

◎ 什么样的人不适合用麦冬？

因为麦冬性质略偏寒凉，而且有养阴润肺作用，因此外感风寒咳嗽、平素怕冷喜暖、胃寒喜饮热水、大便溏薄者不适合服用麦冬。

若服用麦冬后出现怕冷、胃寒、腹泻者应该停用，可适当服用生姜水缓解症状。

【 广医专家话食疗 】

◎ 麦冬食疗用法用量

麦冬药性甘润和缓，日常代茶饮或居家佐餐如煲汤、煮粥等，可以用10~15g。

◎ 麦冬最适合什么季节服用？

麦冬四季皆可服用，因为其具有润肺、清心的作用，所以尤其适合于夏、秋季节服用。

◎ 如何搭配药材、食材？

麦冬甘寒滋润，取其养阴疗效时，尤其是滋补肺阴时常佐入白砂糖或蜂蜜等增强其养阴润燥的功效；治疗肺阴不足，干咳少痰或痰中带血，手脚心烦热，盗汗等，常与天冬、玉竹、百合、生地黄等合用。

煮粥时常可搭配绿豆、薏苡仁等清热健脾；煲汤时常可搭配乌鸡、玉竹、枸杞子等滋阴润燥。

◎ 麦冬、沙参食疗时如何选择？

麦冬与沙参都是甘寒之品，均入肺胃二经，具有清肺养阴、清热生津的食疗功效，常搭配使用，可互相提高疗效。与沙参相比麦冬还能清心安神，因此如有虚烦失眠、心慌多梦更为适宜。此外，麦冬还可用于热病津伤、肠燥便秘。南沙参有祛痰之功，津伤燥咳痰黏更宜。

## 小验方

1. 治疗心热烦闷，口渴，舌红少津

    麦冬 15g，鲜竹叶 10g，粟米 100g。麦冬、竹叶煎水取汁，粟米加水煮至半熟时加入前汁，再煮至粥熟。每次服粥 100g，每日 1 次。

2. 治疗冠心病心绞痛

    麦冬 45g，加水煎取 30~40ml，分次服用，连服 3~18 个月。

3. 治疗肠燥便秘，大便干结

    麦冬 15g，生地黄 15g，玄参 15g。水煎服，每日 1 剂。

# 六、五味子

## 【广医药师谈选药】

◎ 五味子的产地主要在哪里？

五味子为木兰科植物五味子的干燥成熟果实；主产于东北，习称"北五味子"。

◎ 五味子如何炮制与保存？

于通风干燥处贮藏。生用或经醋、蜜拌蒸晒干用。

◎ 五味子生用、醋制和蜜制使用有什么区别？

五味子饮片分为生五味子、醋五味子和蜜五味子，生用生津止渴作用强，醋五味子敛肺止咳力优，蜜五味子益气养心作用好。


## 【广医医师说功效】

◎ 药性与功效——收敛固涩、益气生津、补肾宁心

五味子味道酸甘，中医认为酸味的中药具有收敛固涩的作用，其药性偏温，又能够生津止渴；五味子入肺、心、肾经而补益这些脏腑的不足，因此该药还有敛肺止咳、补肾益精、养心宁神的作用。此外，五味子还能收涩止泻，止汗止遗。

◎ 适用人群——气阴虚体质，久病虚喘、遗精滑精、久泻下利、津伤口渴

五味子主要适用于气阴虚的人群，尤其是肺、心、肾久病虚损的患者。多用于久病虚喘、自汗盗汗、津伤口渴、心慌心悸、遗精滑精、腰膝酸软、不孕不育、久泻不止、失眠多梦等属气阴亏虚者。

肺虚咳喘为主者，多见久病咳嗽，咳痰，气喘、活动后明显，乏力，胸闷等。

津伤消渴为主者，多见发热、心烦、口渴欲饮、饮不解渴、口咽干等。

久泻不止为主者，多见脘腹胀满、纳差、食后胸膈不适、下利清谷、完谷不化、五更泻泄等。

遗精滑精为主者，多见腰膝酸软、精液清冷、阳痿早泄、不育不孕等。

◎ 适用病证

五味子可用于哮喘、腹泻、肝功能损伤、心律不齐、高血压、不育不孕、老年痴呆、帕金森病等疾病见气阴两虚证候的治疗。

◎ 什么样的人不适合用五味子？

五味子性质略偏温，以收涩为功，因此有外感、痰湿、湿热、瘀血、食积等实证者不宜使用，平素表现为恶寒、发热、痰多、舌红苔厚腻、小便黄、大便干等患者应慎用。

【 广医专家话食疗 】

◎ 五味子食疗用法用量

五味子药性酸甘收涩，日常代茶饮可以用1~3g。

◎ 五味子最适合什么季节服用？

五味子四季皆可服用，因为其具有收敛的作用，尤其适合于秋季、冬季服用。

◎ 如何搭配药材、食材？

五味子酸甘收涩，取其敛肺止咳，治疗久病虚喘时，常可与山茱萸、熟地黄、山药等同用；配伍麻黄、细辛、干姜等还可治疗外寒里饮证的咳嗽。治疗自汗、盗汗时，可与黄芪、麻黄根、浮小麦、牡蛎等同用。本品能补肾涩精止遗，为治肾虚精关不固遗精、滑精之常用药，可与桑螵蛸、龙骨、菟丝子、覆盆子、山茱萸、熟地黄、山药等同用。治脾肾虚寒久泻不止，可与吴茱萸、补骨脂、肉豆蔻等同用。治热伤气阴，汗多口渴者，常与人参、麦冬、山药、知母、天花粉等同用。

煮粥时常可搭配芡实、白扁豆、山药等健脾补肾；煲汤时常可搭配乌鸡、甲鱼、海参等补肾益精。

◎ 南、北五味子食疗时如何选择？

南、北五味子功效上区别不大，一般代茶饮均可使用。北五味子补肾效果好，若是肾虚精关不固，以遗精、滑精、腰膝酸软、阳痿早泄、不育不孕等为主时，以北五味子为宜。

## 小验方

### 1. 治疗失眠健忘

鲈鱼 1 条，五味子 50g，料酒、精盐、葱段、姜片、胡椒粉、生油各适量。将五味子浸泡洗净。将鲈鱼去鳞、鳃、内脏，洗净放入锅内，再放入料酒、盐、葱、姜、生油、清水、五味子，煮至鱼肉熟、浓汤成，拣去葱姜，用胡椒粉调味即成。每周 1 剂，分数次食用，用量不限。

### 2. 治疗性欲减退，夜尿频数

菟丝子 100g，五味子 50g，低度白酒 100ml。将菟丝子、五味子淘净、晒干，同入酒瓶中，加酒后密封瓶口，每日振摇 1 次，浸泡 10 天后开始饮用。每日 2 次，每次 15ml。

### 3. 治疗久病虚咳

五味子 250g，加水适量，煎熬取汁，浓缩成稀膏，加等量或适量蜂蜜，以小火煎沸，待冷备用。每次服 1~2 匙，空腹时沸水冲服。

# 七、芦荟

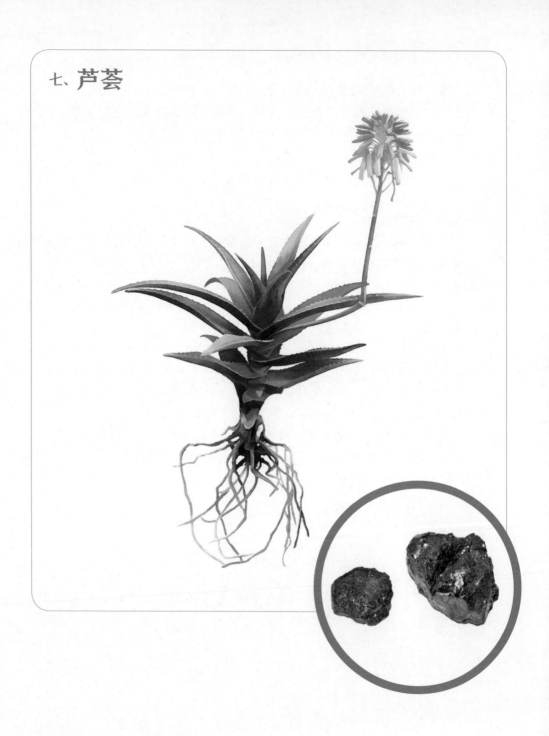

◎ 芦荟的人药部位是哪里?

　　为百合科植物库拉索芦荟、好望角芦荟或其他同属近缘植物叶的汁液浓缩干燥物。

◎ 芦荟的主要产地有哪些?

　　早在唐代,芦荟便由伊朗传入中国。现如今斑纹芦荟是中国特有品种,主要种植于福建、台湾、广东、广西、四川、云南等地。

◎ 如何储存芦荟?

　　将芦荟放置阴凉通风处,避光储存。

【 广医医师说功效 】

◎ 药性与功效——清肝泻火、泻下通便、杀虫疗疳

　　芦荟性味苦、寒,入肝、大肠经,寒能除热,苦能燥湿泻热,亦能杀虫。入肝经,泻肝经实火,治疗由于肝火盛导致的便秘溲赤、头晕头痛、烦躁易怒。入大肠经,泻下通便,用于热结便秘。

◎ 适用人群——肝火旺盛

　　芦荟对强体质(中医谓之实证型)的人较为适宜。患有高血压、便秘,或精力旺盛、红脸膛、易上火者都属此类。

　　肝火旺盛为主者,临床表现主要有头晕胀痛,且疼痛较为剧烈,还有面红目赤、口苦口干、急躁易怒、耳鸣如潮、小便短黄、大便秘结,以及舌红苔黄、脉弦数等表现。

◎ 适用病证

　　芦荟主要适用于热结便秘、头痛、目赤惊风、虫积腹痛、疥癣、痔瘘等属肝火旺盛证者。

◎ 什么样的人不适合用芦荟？

芦荟性味苦、寒，药理研究证明，芦荟中含有芦荟大黄素等蒽醌衍生物，在体内分解后会引起消化道的不良反应，所以孕妇及脾胃虚寒作泻的小儿禁用。

【广医专家话食疗】

◎ 芦荟食疗用法用量

内服：入丸、散，0.5~1.5g。外用：适量，研末调敷。作为蔬菜食用的新鲜芦荟一般常规用量为每天 15g 左右。

◎ 芦荟最适合什么季节服用？

芦荟四季皆可服用。在夏天摄入芦荟可以减少身体对食物中油脂的吸收，达到减重和排毒的目的。

◎ 如何搭配药材、食材？

芦荟治疗肝经实火证见躁狂易怒、惊悸抽搐等症，常与龙胆、黄芩、黄柏、黄连、大黄、当归等同用。治疗蛔虫腹痛，可与使君子、苦楝皮等配合应用。鲜芦荟的食用方法有生食、凉拌、榨汁等，但是老人、儿童以及对芦荟过敏者不宜食用。

◎ 芦荟、番泻叶食疗时如何选择？

芦荟与番泻叶皆能泻下通便，擅于治疗热结便秘，但是芦荟擅长清泄肝热，同时可用于小儿疳积。而番泻叶则擅长泻下导滞，且又能行水消胀，治疗腹水肿胀等症。

小验方

1. 治疗便秘

每晚睡前取芦荟鲜叶 5g，蜂蜜 30g，开水冲服，可缓解便秘。

2. 治疗小儿疳积

取使君子、芦荟叶各等份，晒干，研细粉，米汤调服，每次 3~6g。

### 3. 治疗烧伤

根据烧伤面积取新鲜芦荟叶片洗净，剥去表皮后取其胶冻部分，敷于经清洁消毒的烧伤部位，然后用消毒纱布覆盖固定。烧伤当天每1~3小时换药1次，以后每日换药2~3次。一般1~3小时内疼痛即可减轻或消失，红肿逐渐消退。经2~8天痊愈，不留疤痕。

# 八、石斛

◎ 石斛的入药部位是哪里？

为新鲜或干燥的茎。

◎ 石斛的主要产地有哪些？

长江以南各地均有栽培石斛，尤以安徽、浙江、云南、贵州、广东、广西等地最为著名。

◎ 石斛如何储存？

石斛应于常温（20℃以下）、避光、干燥、通风处保存。也可以放在3~5℃的冰箱冷藏保存，可存放 3~6 个月。

【 广医医师说功效 】

◎ 药性与功效——益胃生津、滋阴清热

石斛甘能滋养，微寒清凉，以清滋为用。入胃经，能养胃阴、生津液；入肾经，能滋肾阴、清虚热。适用于口渴唇燥或中暑后耗津过多，口干舌红，低热不退等病症。

◎ 适用人群——热盛伤津、胃阴不足

石斛主要用于热盛伤津、胃阴不足者。

热盛伤津为主者，多见舌苔黄、发热、口渴喜饮等。

胃阴不足为主者，多见痞满、呕吐、呃逆为主要症状，还伴有口燥、咽干、舌红、少苔、脉细数等。

◎ 适用病证

石斛可用于治疗慢性咽炎、血栓闭塞性脉管炎、关节炎、皮肤化脓性感染等疾病的治疗。

◎ 什么样的人不适合用石斛?

石斛具有益胃生津、滋阴清热的功效,因此阳虚有寒、温热病、湿温尚未化燥者不应服用,严重者可能加重病情。孕妇应在医师指导下服用,避免过量服用。

## 【 广医专家话食疗 】

◎ 石斛食疗用法用量

石斛饮片药用一般为 6~12g,鲜品 15~30g。过量食用石斛可对人体造成伤害,因此健康以及亚健康人群用药干品应控制在 3~5g,鲜品则控制在 10~20g。

◎ 石斛最适合什么季节服用?

石斛最适宜冬季服用。每年 12 月到翌年 2 月是石斛的采收季节,此时的石斛营养及药用价值最高。石斛具有滋阴生津的功效,冬季气温低,天气干燥,石斛可帮助滋养脏腑、缓解干燥。

◎ 如何搭配药材、食材?

石斛配合天花粉、麦冬、沙参、山药、玉竹等,可用于治疗胃有虚寒者;与南沙参、枇杷叶、生地黄、麦冬、百合、秦艽、银柴胡、忍冬藤等配合食用可以治疗虚热口干、虚汗多等症状。石斛与冬虫夏草、水鸭等一起熬汤,可养胃阴、滋肾阴、润肺、补脾;与猪肉、生姜、麦冬等搭配,可以清胃热、生津止渴、滋肾清热、明目。

◎ 石斛、玉竹食疗时如何选择?

石斛与玉竹都能养阴,但玉竹味甘多液,具有补虚清热、生津止渴的功效。而石斛则能够滋阴清热、养胃健脾、止烦渴、降胃火,达到清中有补、补中有清的效果。

**治疗肝火上炎型高血压**

　　石斛 15g（先煎），石决明 30g（先煎），桑寄生 15g，决明子 10g。水煎服，每日 1 剂，分 2 次服用。

# 九、红花

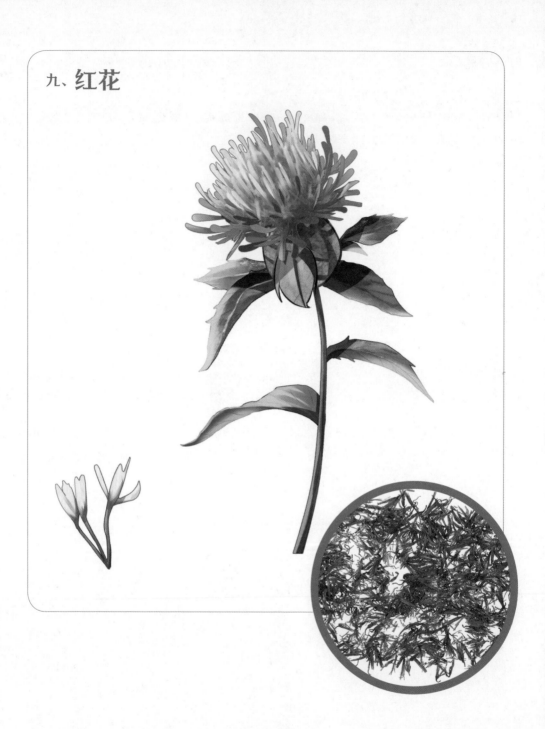

◎ 红花的入药部位是哪里？

菊科植物红花的干燥花。

◎ 红花的主要产地有哪些？

红花原产地在伊朗、西班牙等国。此外，中国河南、江苏、上海等地有引种栽培，现中国红花最大产地在新疆。

◎ 红花如何储存？

红花应置阴凉干燥处，防潮、防蛀。若发现受潮，要及时开箱晾晒或微火烘干，待热气发散凉透后再装箱密封保存，注意不可暴晒。

◎ 如何挑选质量好的红花？

以表面红黄色或者红色，颜色鲜艳，花蕊为圆柱形，顶端微微分叉，泡入水中为橙红色、闻之有淡香味，摸之柔软，味微苦者为佳。

【广医医师说功效】

◎ 药性与功效——活血散瘀，通经止痛

红花性温味辛，归肝、心经，可活血通经、散瘀止痛。其色赤苦温，专入心肝血分，属行散之品，少用可活血，多用可行血。因此擅治瘀血诸症。

◎ 适用人群——瘀血体质、月经不调

红花可用于治疗妇女痛经、闭经以及产后腹痛，同时适用于各种瘀血症状，跌打损伤，冠心病等疾病。凡体内有瘀血者可在医师指导下服用。

瘀血体质者，多见脸色暗沉，舌质紫暗或有瘀点，苔薄白或薄黄，脉涩或弦等，妇女月经量少、色暗、有血块。

◎ 适用病证

红花可用于治疗外伤、闭塞性脑血管疾病、冠心病、心肌梗死、脉管炎等疾病，对高脂血症、糖尿病并发症、月经不调、类风湿关节炎等有辅助治疗作用。

◎ 什么样的人不适合用红花？

有凝血功能障碍、有出血倾向者，不宜食用红花。平素月经量较多或妊娠期妇女也应慎用。

【 广医专家话食疗 】

◎ 红花食疗用法用量

红花内服煎汤一般用 3~10g，养血活血可用 3~5g 泡水，活血祛瘀用 6~10g，代茶饮。

◎ 红花最适合什么季节服用？

红花一年四季均可食用。

◎ 如何搭配药材、食材？

红花配桃仁：红花辛散温通，功能活血祛瘀、通经止痛；桃仁甘润苦降性平，功能活血祛瘀、润肠通便。两药相合，相得益彰，活血祛瘀力增强，凡瘀血证均可服用。

红花与大枣、桃仁、当归、陈皮泡水，可以有效改善因气血两虚导致的面色淡白、倦怠乏力，以及女性月经量少、色淡等症状；与生姜、白芍、蜂蜜、桑叶合用代茶饮，可以缓解瘀血闭阻经络而导致的关节疼痛、腰背酸痛等症状。

◎ 红花、藏红花食疗时如何选择？

藏红花是一种名贵的中药材，两者虽然名字相似，但功效有所不同，藏红花具有活血化瘀、凉血解毒、安神的功效，可以治疗闭经、产后瘀阻、忧郁苦闷、惊悸发狂等相关病症。而红花具有活血通经、消肿止痛的功效，活血力度不如藏红花。

1. 治疗痛经

   红花 6g，鸡血藤 30g，加水煎取汁，加适量黄酒，一次服下。

2. 治疗关节炎肿痛

   红花炒过后研成粉末，加入等量的地瓜粉，用盐水或白酒调好，涂敷患处。

# 十、天麻

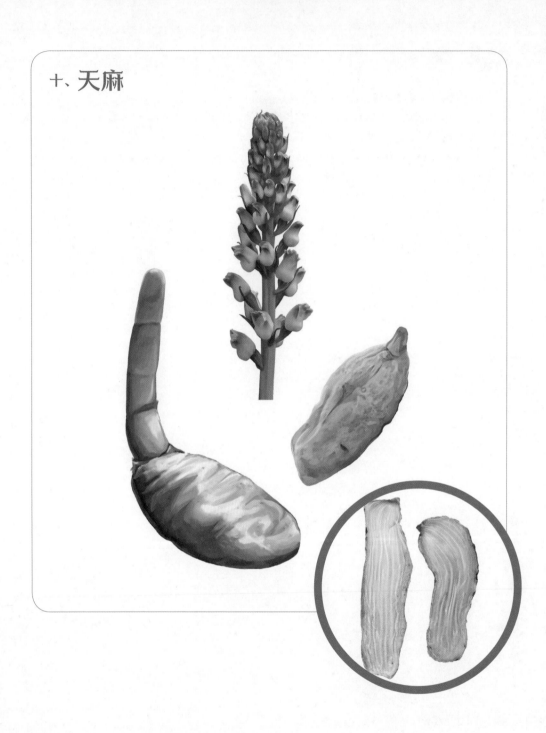

## 【广医药师谈选药】

◎ 天麻入药用的是哪部分？

以兰科植物天麻的干燥块茎入药。

◎ 哪里产的天麻好？

云南昭通产的天麻质量较好。

◎ 如何辨别天麻质量的好坏？

以角质样、切面半透明、色黄白者为佳。

◎ 天麻如何保存？

新鲜天麻可用水轻轻冲净泥，晒干水分，用报纸加塑料袋密封放入冰箱冷藏保存。刚挖出的天麻不能刮伤，放入箱子，一层天麻一层沙子，盖上薄膜，不密封，置于10℃左右干燥处储存。干天麻放入玻璃瓶密封好放阴凉通风处保存，不可冷冻储存，否则易变质。

◎ 天麻冬产和春产有什么区别？

天麻主要分为冬麻和春麻，冬麻外观饱满，皱纹细小，色黄白，不易折断，品质更佳。春麻皱纹粗大，色灰褐，易折断，品质较差。

## 【广医医师说功效】

◎ 药性与功效——息风止痉、平抑肝阳、祛风通络

天麻味甘性平，归肝经，具有息风止痉、平抑肝阳、祛风通络的功效。天麻擅于息风止痉，治疗多种肝风病证，内风外风均可治疗，又能平抑肝阳，治疗肝阳上亢病证。

◎ 适用人群——外风侵袭，肝风内动，肝阳上亢

天麻主要治疗肝风内动、肝阳上亢的人群。多用于头痛、眩晕，以及

感受风邪、四肢痉挛、小儿惊风者。

感受外风为主者，多见风湿痹痛、关节屈伸不利、筋骨疼痛等。

肝风内动为主者，多见眩晕昏仆、惊痫抽搐、小儿惊风等。

肝阳上亢为主者，多见头痛眩晕、面红目赤、急躁易怒、心烦失眠等。

◎ 适用病证

天麻可用于高血压、眩晕、抽搐、风湿痹痛、失眠等疾病证属肝阳上亢者。

◎ 什么样的人不适合用天麻？

血虚、阴津亏损、血压较低者慎用天麻。

【 广医专家话食疗 】

◎ 天麻食疗用法用量

天麻味甘性平，可以配合其他食材用于蒸、煮、炖，一天用量不宜超过 40g。

◎ 天麻最适合什么季节服用？

天麻四季皆可服用，因其滋补性较强，冬季服用效果更佳。

◎ 如何搭配药材、食材？

治疗小儿急惊风时，可配伍僵蚕、全蝎、钩藤等；治疗小儿脾虚慢惊风，可与僵蚕、人参、白术合用；治疗小儿诸惊，可与制天南星、全蝎、僵蚕合用；治疗角弓反张、破伤风等，可与防风、天南星、白附子配合使用；治疗肝阳上亢所致的头晕，可配合石决明、钩藤、牛膝；治疗中风肢体麻木、手足不遂时，常配伍秦艽、羌活、桑枝、没药、制乌头等。

在日常炒菜时常搭配猪肉起到滋补作用；与粳米一起熬粥，具有平肝息风、行气活血功效。

**小验方**

**治疗头晕、目眩**

天麻 30g，鸡蛋 3 个，水 1 000ml，同煮，鸡蛋熟后食用。

# 十一、地黄

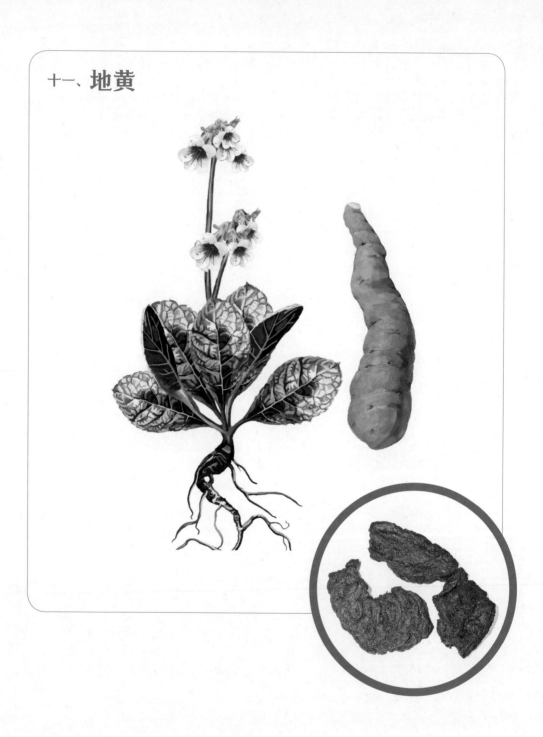

◎ 地黄入药用的是哪部分？

以玄参科植物地黄的干燥块根入药。

◎ 哪里产的地黄好？

以河南产的地黄质量较好。

◎ 如何辨别地黄质量的好坏？

地黄根据炮制方法不同分为生地黄和熟地黄，生地黄以切面乌黑者为佳，熟地黄以块肥大、断面乌黑色、味甜者为佳。

◎ 地黄如何保存？

熟地黄可密封好放在干燥阴凉处保存，隔绝空气和水分，以防变质。熟地黄也可以密封后放入冰箱冷冻保存，延长储存时间。生地黄可以切片晒干密封后放在干燥阴凉处保存，或放入冰箱冷藏。

◎ 生地黄和熟地黄有什么区别？

地黄饮片分为生地黄和熟地黄两种。生地黄是鲜地黄除掉芦头、须根、泥沙，烘焙到约八成干而成；熟地黄是生地黄用酒炖至酒吸尽，晾晒到表面黏液稍干，切成块或厚片，干燥备用。生地黄味甘性寒，以清热凉血、养阴生津为主，熟地黄味甘、微温，以补血滋阴、益精填髓为主。

【广医医师说功效】

◎ 药性与功效——生地黄：清热凉血、养阴生津；熟地黄：补血滋阴、益精填髓

生地黄甘、寒，归心、肝、肾经，入营、血分，擅于清热凉血，多用于治疗温热病热入营血导致的发斑、神昏谵语等，还可治疗血热出血。因其性寒、质地甘润，可以养阴生津，治疗烦渴、骨蒸潮热等阴虚病症。

熟地黄甘、微温，归肝、肾经。以补血滋阴为主要功效，擅于益精填髓，是治疗血虚诸症之要药。主治肝肾阴虚证。

◎ 适用人群——生地黄：热入营血、血热出血、阴虚、发热；熟地黄：血虚诸症、肝肾不足

**生地黄**适用于热入血分、出血、伤阴病证者。

热入营血为主者，多见壮热烦渴、神昏舌绛、发斑发疹、谵语等。

血热出血为主者，多见吐血、衄血、便血、崩漏、尿血、产后出血等。

阴虚、发热为主者，多见心烦、口渴多饮、骨蒸潮热、夜热早凉、肠燥便秘等。

**熟地黄**适用于阴血亏虚、肝肾不足者。

血虚诸习正为主者，可见面色萎黄、心悸失眠、眩晕、崩漏、月经不调等。

肝肾不足为主者，可见腰膝酸软、耳鸣、耳聋、遗精盗汗、消渴、骨蒸潮热、须发早白、五迟（立、行、语、发、齿迟）、五软（头、口、手、足、肌肉软）。

◎ 适用病证

生地黄可用于治疗血热出血、骨蒸潮热等属阴虚血热证者；熟地黄可用于治疗骨质疏松、心悸失眠、耳鸣等属肝肾不足证者。

◎ 什么样的人不适合用地黄？

生地黄性寒，脾虚湿滞、腹满便溏者不宜服用；熟地黄较为滋腻碍胃，不易消化，湿盛、气滞、痰多、中满者忌服，若必须服用，可配伍砂仁、陈皮。

【广医专家话食疗】

◎ 地黄食疗用法用量

地黄每日用量一般为 10~30g，可用来煲汤、熬粥、炖肉等。

◎ 地黄最适合什么季节服用？

一年四季均可服用。因为地黄甘润，适合养阴，"春夏养阳，秋冬养阴"，因此秋冬季节服用更为适合。

◎ 如何搭配药材、食材？

生地黄味甘性寒，可搭配连翘、玄参、黄连等治疗壮热、神昏、烦渴舌绛者；搭配赤芍、牡丹皮、水牛角治疗发斑、神昏谵语等；与大青叶、水牛角同用治疗热毒炽盛、发斑发疹、颜色紫暗；与侧柏叶、地榆、槐花、小蓟、茜草搭配治疗出血证；配伍沙参、麦冬等治疗烦渴多饮；搭配地骨皮、知母、麦冬、青蒿、鳖甲治疗骨蒸潮热、夜热早凉等。

熟地黄质润、微温，可搭配白芍、当归、川芎治疗血虚诸症；搭配山茱萸、山药、知母等治疗肝肾阴虚诸症；搭配何首乌、牛膝等治疗须发早白；搭配狗脊、锁阳、龟甲等治疗五迟五软。

日常生活中，生地黄可搭配枸杞子、乌鸡养阴生津，治疗盗汗、腰酸背痛；搭配猪瘦肉、百合等煲汤，养心除烦，宁心安神。熟地黄可炖鸡滋补气血，还可搭配羊肉煲汤助阳生发。

## 小验方

1. 治疗腰膝酸软、耳鸣

熟地黄 50g，猪蹄 1 只，杜仲 30g，枸杞子 30g，怀牛膝 30g。炖煮，当餐食用。

2. 治疗干咳、咽干、口渴等

熟地黄 40g，去核大枣 6 枚，冬虫夏草 10g，鸭肉 500g，前三者放入老鸭腹中，加水，小火隔水炖 3 小时，当餐食用。

3. 治疗功能性子宫出血

生地黄、当归各 30g，羊肉 250g，盐适量，煲汤食用。

4. 治疗蝴蝶斑

生地黄 100g，枸杞子 30g，怀山药 200g，白鸭 500g。用葱、姜、调味品等腌白鸭后与药同蒸，当餐食用。

# 第三节
## 名贵中药

### 一、人参

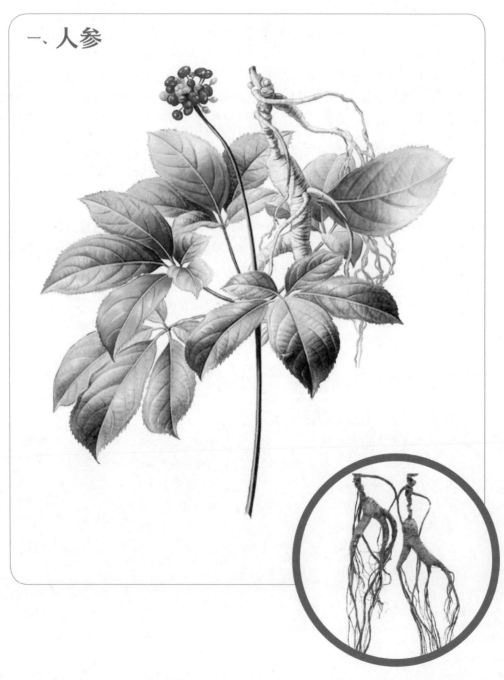

◎ **人参入药用哪部分？**

为五加科植物人参的根与根茎入药。

◎ **哪里产的人参最好？**

吉林抚松人参产量大，质量好，称为"吉林参"。

◎ **人参的各种品名代表什么意思？**

野生人参名"山参"；栽培人参称"园参"。园参一般应栽培 6~7 年后收获。

鲜参洗净后干燥者称"生晒参"；人参蒸制后干燥者称"红参"；人参加工时断下的细根称"参须"。山参经晒干称"生晒山参"。

◎ **如何挑选山参？**

山参以支大、芦长、体灵、皮细、色嫩黄、纹细密、饱满、无破伤者为佳，支头大者为上品。

◎ **山参、红参、生晒参、参须应用有何不同？**

山参大补元气，为参中之上品；红参补气中带有刚健温燥之性，长于振奋阳气；生晒参性较平和，适用于扶正祛邪；参须效力较小而缓和。

【 广医医师说功效 】

◎ **药性与功效——大补元气、补脾益肾、生津、安神**

人参味甘、性微温，大补元气，能回阳气于垂绝，是治疗虚劳内伤第一要药，所以凡是大失血、大汗、大吐泻以及一切疾病导致的元气虚极欲脱之证，单用人参一味药就十分有效。人参入脾经，可以补脾调中，鼓舞脾气，以助运化，输布津液，以达生津止渴之效。另外，人参大补元气，气足则神旺，故有安神之效。

◎ 适用人群——元气虚脱，肺脾气虚、热病伤津

人参主要适用于元气大虚，气虚津伤者。多用于失血与疮疡溃后，气血俱虚，面色苍白，恶寒发热，手足发凉，自汗或出冷汗，脉微细欲绝者。

元气虚脱为主者，多见面色苍白、呼吸短促、四肢乏力、头晕、手足发凉、脉微细欲绝等。

肺脾气虚为主者，多见不思饮食、大便溏薄、精神不振、形体消瘦、肢体倦怠、少气懒言、自汗畏风、易感外邪、面色萎黄或白，或肢体浮肿、舌淡苔白、脉缓软无力等。

热病伤津为主者，多见体倦乏力、精神不振、心悸气短、干咳少痰、喉干、舌绛、渴饮不止、大便干结等。

◎ 适用病证

人参可用于因大汗、大泻、大失血或大病、久病所致元气虚极欲脱、气短神疲、脉微欲绝的重危人群，或脾胃虚弱、食欲不振之人，或热病后期、口渴乏力、多汗、脉虚弱者的治疗。

◎ 什么样的人不适合用人参？

因为人参是一种补气药，如没有气虚症状而随便服用，是不适宜的。尤其是体质壮实的人，并无虚弱征象，则不必进服补药。妄用人参，如误用或多用，往往导致胸闷腹胀等症。

另外，服用人参后忌吃萝卜，忌饮茶。

【广医专家话食疗】

◎ 人参食疗用法用量

人参药性甘温微苦，日常代茶饮可以用 5~15g。居家佐餐如炖菜、煲汤、煮粥等，饮片可以用 10~20g。

◎ 人参最适合什么季节服用？

人参药性甘温微苦，日常服用一定要注意季节变化。一般来说，秋冬

季节天气凉爽，较宜进食；而夏季天气炎热，则不宜食用。

◎ 如何搭配药材、食材？

人参大补元气，复脉固脱，单用一味药即有效，如独参汤。若气虚欲脱兼见汗出，四肢逆冷者，与附子同用，以补气固脱、回阳救逆；若气虚欲脱兼见汗出身暖，渴喜冷饮，舌红干燥者，常与麦冬、五味子配伍，以补气养阴；脾虚不运，常与白术、茯苓、黄芪、当归同用；热伤气津者，常与知母、石膏同用。

在日常炖菜、煲汤时，常与粳米、瘦肉、鸡、鸭、鱼等食材搭配，起到滋补强身的功效。

◎ 人参、西洋参食疗时如何选择？

人参与西洋参都有补气作用，但人参补气作用比西洋参更佳。西洋参性寒，具有补气养阴、泻火除烦、养胃生津的功效。所以人参更适用于久病气虚的人群，而西洋参则适用于气阴两虚有热之人。

**小验方**

1. **治疗食欲不振，自汗易感**
   人参10g，粳米100g，熬粥，每日早、晚各1次温服。
2. **治疗神疲乏力，烦渴多饮**
   人参6g，鸡蛋1个。人参研末，与鸡蛋清调匀，蒸熟，每日服1次。
3. **治疗面色萎黄，心神不安**
   人参5g，银耳15g。文火熬汤，饮汤食银耳，每日早、晚各1次温服。

# 二、西洋参

◎ 西洋参的药用部位是什么?

以五加科植物西洋参的干燥根入药。

◎ 哪里产的西洋参好?

西洋参通常按产地分成花旗参与加拿大参,两者虽然同种,但因为气候影响,前者的表面横纹比后者更明显,有效成分含量也较高。

◎ 如何辨别西洋参质量的好坏?

优质西洋参主根较短,多呈纺锤形、圆柱形或圆锥形,常有分枝,分叉角度大;外表横纹细密,质轻,粉性少;气香而浓,味微甜带苦,口感清爽,味能久留口中。一般又以野生者为上品,栽培者次之。

◎ 西洋参如何保存?

把选好的西洋参装在一定的容器里,放在通风处进行晾晒,不时翻动,至干为止。

◎ 西洋参和人参药用有何区别?

西洋参性寒,具有补气养阴、泻火除烦、养胃生津等多重功效,多用于肺热燥咳、气虚懒言、四肢倦怠、烦躁易怒、热病后伤阴津液亏损等。人参药性偏温,能大补元气,补益之力强于西洋参,故对虚劳内有火热者不宜。此外,人参尚能补益心肾之气,安神增智,还常用于失眠、健忘、心悸怔忡及肾不纳气之虚喘气短。

【广医医师说功效】

◎ 药性与功效——补气养阴、清火生津

西洋参补益元气、养阴,能补心、肺、脾之气阴。西洋参性凉,尚能清火生津,适用于热伤气津所致身热汗多、口渴心烦、体倦少气、脉虚数者。

◎ 适用人群——气阴两虚，内热津伤

西洋参主要适用于气阴两虚，内热津伤的人群。

气阴两伤为主者，多见于热病或大汗、大泻、耗伤元气及阴津所致神疲乏力，气短息促，自汗热黏，心烦口渴，尿短赤涩，大便干结，舌燥，脉细数无力。

心气阴两虚为主者，多见失眠、多梦、心悸、心痛。

肺气阴两虚为主者，多见短气喘促、咳嗽痰少或痰中带血。

脾气阴两虚为主者，多见纳呆食滞、口渴思饮。

◎ 适用病证

西洋参可用于治疗神疲乏力、心悸失眠、咳嗽喘促等证属气阴两虚者。

◎ 什么样的人不适合用西洋参？

素体脾胃虚寒的人不适合用西洋参，服用西洋参后，一般会出现畏寒、体温下降、食欲不振、腹痛腹泻；也有的女性会发生痛经和经期延迟。

【 广医专家话食疗 】

◎ 西洋参食疗用法用量？

西洋参由于品性温和，适合进补。煮服，3g；炖服，2~5g；蒸服，5g；泡水服用，3~5g。

◎ 西洋参最适合什么季节服用？

西洋参四季皆可服用。与其他参类不同，西洋参是一种"清凉"参，因其具有益气养阴、清火生津之功效，尤其适合夏季"清补"。

◎ 如何搭配药材、食材？

西洋参配麦冬：西洋参益气、养阴生津，麦冬可增强其养阴生津之功。两者配合作代茶饮。用于热病气阴两伤，烦热口渴；或老人气阴虚少，咽干口燥，津液不足，舌干少苔。

煲汤时常与乌鸡、百合、枸杞子等滋阴、清热、生津的食材搭配，起到清热养阴的功效；与川贝、梨、冰糖相配，用于阴虚肺热、咳嗽痰黏、咽干口渴。

◎ 西洋参、人参食疗时如何选择？

人参和西洋参都属于补益类药物，其化学成分相似，具有强身健体、抗疲劳、降血糖、安定精神、提高免疫力等多种生理活性作用。然而食疗药膳中应注意区别对待，素体阳热、容易"上火"之人应选用西洋参，而平素怕冷、虚弱的人则应选用生晒人参。

**小验方**

1. 增强免疫力

    西洋参 3g，切片，代茶饮，频服。

2. 治疗久治难愈之咳嗽

    西洋参 5g，百合 30g，蜂蜜 80g，蒸熟食之。

3. 健脑，增强记忆力

    西洋参 5g，灵芝 10g，煎水服，每日 2 次。

# 三、鹿茸

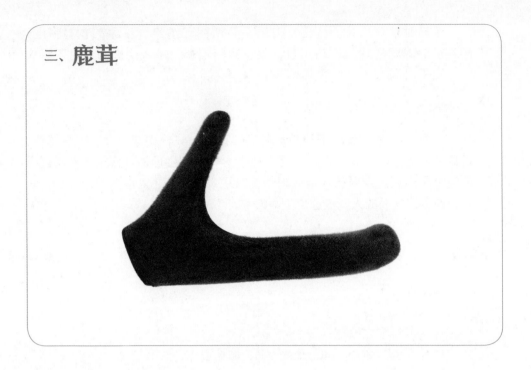

【广医药师谈选药】

◎ 鹿茸药用的是哪部分？

为鹿科动物梅花鹿或马鹿等雄鹿未骨化密生茸毛的幼角。

◎ 如何挑选鹿茸？

以茸体饱满、挺圆、质嫩、毛细、皮色红棕、体轻者为佳。而细、瘦、底部起筋、毛粗糙、体重者为次货。

鹿茸片以毛孔嫩细，红色小片为佳。

◎ 鹿茸如何保存？

鹿茸应在通风、阴凉、干燥处密封保存。还可在鹿茸周围用布包一些花椒以防虫。

◎ 药性与功效——补肾阳、益精血、强筋骨、调冲任、托疮毒

鹿茸甘温补阳，甘咸滋肾，禀纯阳之性，具生发之气，故能补肾阳、益精血。入肝、肾二经，肾主骨，肾气充则筋骨健，故鹿茸亦有强筋骨之效。中医认为肝肾足则冲任调，气血盛则温补内托，故鹿茸有调冲任、托疮毒之效。

◎ 适用人群——虚寒体质，畏寒肢冷、宫冷不孕、五迟五软

鹿茸主要适用于虚寒体质的人群，尤其是肾阳虚衰、肾虚骨弱、冲任虚寒的人群。多用于畏寒肢冷、阳痿早泄、宫冷不孕、小便频数、腰膝酸痛、头晕耳鸣、精神疲乏等。

肾阳虚衰为主者，多见腰膝酸软，畏寒肢冷，阳痿，五更泄泻，精神委靡，动则气喘，小便困难或夜尿频数，脉沉弱等。

肾虚骨弱为主者，多见肌肉松弛，动则自汗，寐则盗汗，睡不安宁，五迟，或鸡胸龟背，舌苔薄白，脉数无力等。

冲任虚寒为主者，多见子宫虚冷、崩漏、带下、产后贫血及宫冷不孕等。

◎ 适用病证

鹿茸主治肾阳不足，精血亏虚；肝肾不足筋骨痿软；妇女冲任虚寒、带脉不固；疮疡久溃不敛，脓汁清稀或阴疽内陷不起等病证。

◎ 什么样的人不适合用鹿茸？

鹿茸味甘、咸，性温，因此凡体格壮实而无需服食的人或食茸过量的人，都容易引起头涨、胸闷或鼻衄等，须立即停药观察，而不可强行续用。

以下四种情况不宜服用鹿茸：①有"五心烦热"症状，属阴虚者；②小便黄赤，咽喉干燥或干痛，不时感到烦渴而具有内热症状者；③经常流鼻血，或女子行经量多，血色鲜红，舌红脉细，属血热证者；④正逢伤风感冒，出现头痛鼻塞、发热畏寒、咳嗽痰多等症状属于外邪正盛者。

◎ 鹿茸食疗用法用量

鹿茸日常炖服每次用量 1~4g，直接含服为 0.5~1g。居家食用以煲汤、研末熬粥、泡酒饮用为佳。

◎ 鹿茸最适合什么季节服用？

鹿茸性热温燥，补肾阳、益精血、强筋骨，尤其适宜冬季服用。

◎ 如何搭配药材、食材？

取其补肾阳、益精血功效，治疗肾阳虚，精血不足，而见畏寒肢冷、阳痿早泄、宫冷不孕、小便频数时单用即可；治疗阳痿不举，可以与山药同浸酒服用；治疗精血耗竭、面色黧黑、耳聋目昏等，可以与当归乌梅膏为丸服用；治疗诸虚百损，五劳七伤，可与人参、黄芪、当归同用。

煲汤时常可搭配鸡、鸭、大枣、枸杞子、莲子、百合、当归、人参；或鹿茸浸入白酒密闭贮存，半月后日取 10ml 饮用。

◎ 鹿茸片、鹿茸粉食疗时如何选择？

鹿茸片、鹿茸粉功用相同，都是鹿茸的加工品，前者为鹿茸切片，后者为鹿茸片研成的粉。二者同样具有补肾阳、益精血、强筋骨、调冲任、托疮毒的功效。但二者服用方法略有不同，鹿茸片多用于泡酒、炖菜、煲汤，或煮后嚼服；而鹿茸粉则适合熬粥服用。

**小验方**

1. 治疗阳痿遗精，小便频数，腰膝酸软
  鹿茸酒：鹿茸 10g，山药 30g，以白酒 500g 浸渍。每次饮 10~20ml。
2. 治疗精血不足，夜尿多，手足不温
  鹿茸蒸蛋：鹿茸粉 0.5g，鸡蛋 2 个。鸡蛋敲破，倾入碗中，放入鹿茸及盐、胡椒粉，一并调匀，蒸熟食。
3. 治疗宫冷不孕
  鹿茸粥：鹿茸片（粉）0.3g，与粳米或小米熬制成粥食用。

# 四、冬虫夏草

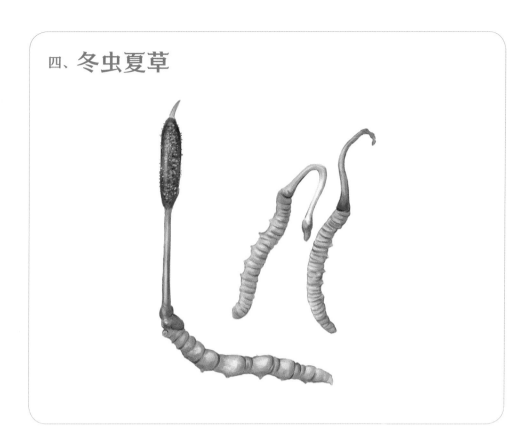

【广医药师谈选药】

◎ 冬虫夏草是虫还是草?

　　冬虫夏草并不是虫,也不是草,而是一种真菌(子囊菌),是麦角菌科真菌冬虫夏草菌寄生在蝙蝠科昆虫幼虫上的子座和幼虫尸体的干燥复合体。冬天时尚保留幼虫的躯壳,夏天则从幼虫躯壳里长出"草"来。所以称为"冬虫夏草"。

◎ 哪里产的冬虫夏草好?

　　冬虫夏草主要生长在中国青海玉树州和果洛州,西藏那曲、昌都、林芝,四川甘孜州一带,以及云南迪庆州。一般认为玉树州和那曲产的虫草质量较优。

◎ 如何辨别冬虫夏草质量的好坏?

　　冬虫夏草虫体似蚕,长约 3~5cm,以虫体完整、丰满肥大,外表色黄亮、内色白，子座短者为佳。冬虫夏草用开水浸泡，虫体变膨大而软，子座颜色变为黑褐色，虫体和子座紧密相连，不脱落。浸出液微有臭味。也可以掰开细看，若有在冬虫夏草中插入铁丝等异物的即是伪劣商品。

◎ 冬虫夏草如何保存？

　　刚买来的冬虫夏草都有些潮而且久置容易发霉、生虫。冬虫夏草储藏要特别注意防潮、防蛀和防虫。如果量很少，而且需要储藏的时间也很短，只需要放在阴凉干燥处即可。如果量大或者需要放置较长时间，最好在储存时放入干燥剂。

◎ 冬虫夏草应该怎么用？

　　用于一般保健，可以将冬虫夏草泡水饮用，而后嚼服；也可以粉碎后装入胶囊服用；还可以用来炖老鸭、蒸猪肉等，或自制虫草酒。


## 【广医医师说功效】


◎ 药性与功效——益肾、补肺、止血化痰

　　冬虫夏草味甘，性质平和，能够益肾补肺，止血化痰，是非常平和的补益人体阴阳的珍贵药物。对于肾虚、肺气虚或肺肾两虚有良好的补益作用，久服也不易引起燥热之象。

◎ 适用人群——气虚、阳虚体质，倦怠乏力、腰痛、遗精，久咳虚喘，咳嗽痰血等

　　冬虫夏草主要适用于肺气虚或者肾阳虚的人群，多用于体质较弱，肾虚腰痛、阳痿遗精，或者久咳虚喘，劳嗽痰血者。

　　肺气虚者，多见平素体虚容易感冒、畏寒自汗，或者干咳少痰、无痰、咳而无力，喘促等。

　　肾虚者，多见腰膝酸软无力、阳痿、遗精、早泄、耳鸣、健忘、神思恍惚，以及肾虚不足、肾不纳气的喘息咳嗽等。

◎ 适用病证

　　冬虫夏草被认为是治疗各种虚损的佳品，可以用于呼吸系统疾病、心

脑血管疾病、肝硬化、肝纤维化等。由于其性平力缓，能平补阴阳，所以也是年老体弱、病后体衰、术后及产后体虚者的调补药食佳品。

◎ 什么样的人不适合用冬虫夏草？

　　冬虫夏草虽然是滋补上品，但并不是人人都适合服用。其主要适合于体虚者，如果平时身体比较壮实，或者有外感发热、湿热内盛，或者患有急性咳嗽、肾功能严重损害的患者，就不适合服用。

## 【广医专家话食疗】

◎ 冬虫夏草食疗用法用量

　　冬虫夏草药性甘平和缓，可单用冬虫夏草每次 2g 研末，空腹送服；日常代茶饮可以用 3~5g。也可用冬虫夏草 5g，配杜仲、续断等，煎汤饮服。

　　居家佐餐如用来炖汤等，则可以用 5~8g。

◎ 冬虫夏草最适合什么季节服用？

　　冬虫夏草四季皆可服用，因其有补肾益肺的作用，特别适合冬季服用。

◎ 如何搭配药材、食材？

　　冬虫夏草味甘性平，取其益肺功效时，常与百合、川贝母、银耳同炖，用于肺结核见咳喘、痰中带血丝的患者；取其益肾功效时，可配狗脊、桑寄生、杜仲、续断等煎汤饮服，用于肾虚腰膝酸软无力等。

　　在日常生活中，常将冬虫夏草与鸡、鸭、牛、羊肉或各种素菜炖服或者用水煎煮服用，可用于诸虚劳损。

### 小验方

1. **平素体虚容易感冒、畏寒自汗**
　　冬虫夏草 5g，老公鸭 1 只，黄酒少许，煮烂食用。
2. **治疗更年期综合征**
　　冬虫夏草 5g，母鸡 1 只，炖汤服用。

# 五、灵芝

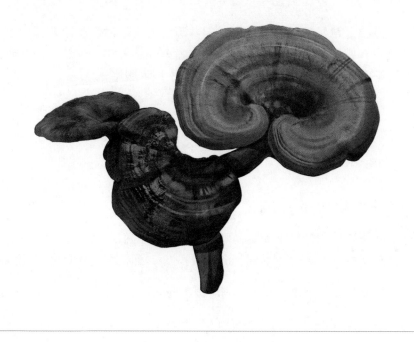

【广医药师谈选药】

◎ 灵芝有多少种，哪种更好？

灵芝品种非常多，有青芝、赤芝、白芝、紫芝等。一般认为赤芝、紫芝药用价值较大。

◎ 如何辨别灵芝质量的好坏？

灵芝的质量可从其形体、色泽、厚薄、比重等方面进行判断。质优的灵芝子实体柄短、肉厚、菌盖的背部或底部用放大镜观察能看到管孔部位，呈淡黄或金黄色为最佳，呈白色的次之，呈灰白色且管孔较大的最次。

◎ 灵芝如何保存？

新鲜的灵芝可以直接食用，但保存期很短。灵芝采收后，去掉表面的泥沙及灰尘，自然晾干或烘干，水分控制在 13% 以下，然后用密封袋包装，放在阴凉干燥处保存。

◎ 如何识别野生灵芝的真假

与人工养殖的灵芝相比，野生灵芝往往色泽更加自然，由于品种不同，常常大小不一，有时子实体下方都会留有不规则虫眼，味道偏苦。

【 广医医师说功效 】

◎ 药性与功效——补气养血、养心安神、止咳平喘

灵芝味甘、微苦，性平，入心、肺、肝、肾经。中医认为甘味药能够起到补益和缓的作用，所以灵芝能够补益人体气血，入心经还能够用于心神不安而养心安神，入肺经还具有止咳平喘的作用。

◎ 适用人群——体虚之人，气血不足、心神不安、咳嗽喘息

灵芝主要适用于体虚的人群，能够补益五脏之气，调节人体免疫力，尤其适宜平素倦怠乏力、饮食量少，或者心悸不安、失眠健忘、神经衰弱、咳喘短气之人，也可用于一般人群的日常保健。

气血不足为主者，多见倦怠乏力、少气懒言、面色㿠白或萎黄、饮食量少等。

心神不安为主者，多见心悸不安、健忘失眠、神经衰弱等。

咳嗽喘息为主者，多见咳嗽无力、喘促、短气、自汗、平素易受风寒等。

◎ 适用病证

灵芝能够提高人体免疫力，可用于高血压、高脂血症、冠心病、白细胞减少症、慢性病毒性肝炎等。

◎ 什么样的人不适合用灵芝?

灵芝是补益气血、延年益寿的佳品，一般人群都可食用。对灵芝过敏者不适合使用。此外，实证患者，平素容易上火、精力旺盛者也不适宜使用。

◎ 灵芝食疗用法用量

灵芝药性甘平和缓，日常代茶饮可以用 5~15g。也可用来煲汤、煮粥、制成灵芝药酒等。

◎ 灵芝最适合什么季节服用？

灵芝性平和，一年四季皆可服用。

◎ 如何搭配药材、食材？

灵芝用于气血不足时，常配合黄芪、当归等；用于心悸失眠时，常配合大枣、莲子心、百合等；用于咳嗽喘时，常配合人参、百合、沙参等。

灵芝作食疗时可单独切片泡水代茶饮；也可煮粥、煲汤时搭配瘦肉、莲子、百合等补益，清心安神；还可以制成灵芝酒，用于神经衰弱、失眠、消化不良、咳嗽气喘、老年性支气管炎等症。

### 小验方

**1. 治疗脾虚气弱，饮食减少，消瘦乏力**

灵芝 30g，仔鸡 1 只。将灵芝及生姜、胡椒、盐、酒放入鸡腹，并加适量的水，蒸至鸡烂熟。饮汤食鸡。

**2. 治疗神经衰弱**

灵芝 6~9g，水煎代茶饮，睡前服。

# Chinese
# Materia Medica

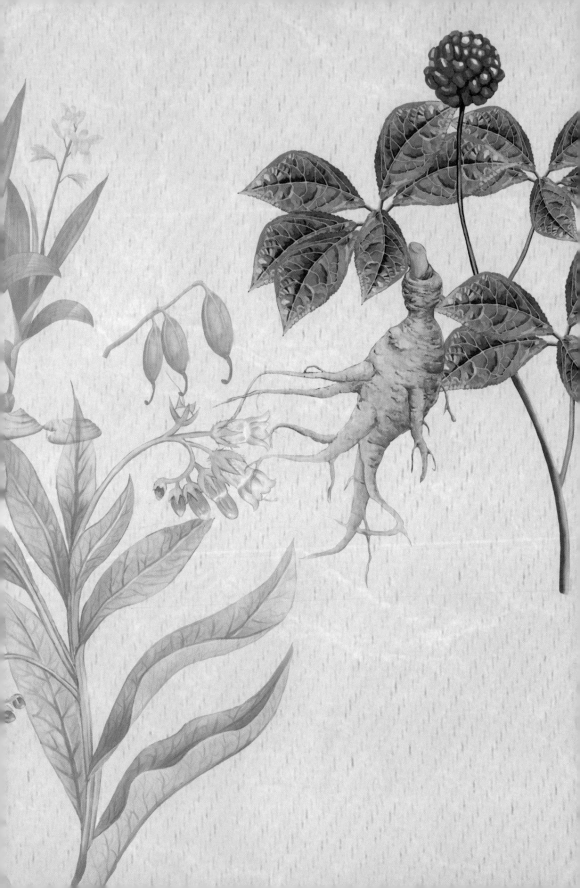

# Chapter 1

# General Knowledge of

# Chinese Medicinals

# Section 1

## Origin, Development, and Cultural Connotation of Chinese Medicinals

Chinese materia medica has a long history. In ancient times, our ancestors relied on the wild to get food and often came into contact with various herbs, which we usually call Chinese medicinals. Some of them are poisonous or even highly toxic. Still, after thousands of practices, the efficacy or toxicity of these medicines has been passed down by word of mouth, and our ancestors gradually accumulated experience in distinguishing medicines from food. In ancient times, when humans slept rough, nine out of ten people got sick, and some animals and plants they ate inadvertently could relieve the related symptoms, which is the early discovery of medicines. Thus, the primitive origin of Chinese medicinals is based on life practice. With the development of human civilization, the creation and use of characters, and the invention of brew and soup, people found under rational thinking that different medicines have distinct effects and, at the same time, diverse eating and processing methods also play an essential intervening role in the efficacy of Chinese medicinals. The earliest extant herbal monograph in China is *Shennong's Classic of Materia Medica*, which contains 365 kinds of medicinals, and is divided into three categories (superior, middle, and inferior) according to their efficacy and effects on the human body. Although the author of *Shennong's Classic of Materia Medica* is unknown and the age of its completion is inconclusive, we can be sure that the classification method of the superior, middle, and inferior categories in this book reveals the basic understanding of medicines in the early days. Meanwhile, at that time, people realized the four natures and five flavors of medicinals, the concerted application, and the classification of preparations. We cannot help but praise that in ancient China, thousands of years ago, the understanding of Chinese medicinals reached such a sophisticated level. Through the development over dynasties, the related research of Chinese medicinals has become a discipline with an integrated system, complete framework, and rich connotation.

Chinese materia medica culture is a crucial branch and an essential component of traditional Chinese medicine (TCM) culture, and it is also a precious historical wealth of Chinese culture. Chinese materia medica culture embodies both ancient medical thinking and vibrant philosophical ideas, which is also the core component deeply rooted in the connotation of our national culture. After invoking the laws of nature and observing many phenomena, the ancients discovered different effects of medicinals based on clinical practice and their unique thinking mode of TCM. For example, red medicinals enter the heart, cyan medicinals enter the liver, yellow medicinals enters the spleen, white medicinal enter the lung, black medicinals enter the kidney, clear flowers and leaves often treat diseases in upper jiao, and heavy seeds, ores, and shells often treat diseases in lower jiao. It is this unique mode of thinking that has guided the clinical application of Chinese medicinals and has protected the health of the Chinese nation for thousands of years. Chinese materia medica is a bright treasure in ancient Chinese medical culture. China and other countries in the world have carried out clinical and basic research on many Chinese medicinals. These studies have all verified the ancient Chinese medicalists' understanding of the efficacy of Chinese medicinals and further promoted the prosperous development of Chinese medicinals. Focusing on the contemporary era, in the process of fighting severe acute respiratory syndrome (SARS) and novel coronavirus infection (COVID-19), Chinese medicinals has played an important role in strengthening the body and eliminating pathogens. It has a significant effect on intervening in severe transformation, shortening the time of conversion, and improving the cure rate. With the change of people's understanding of health and the growing demand for healthcare, TCM has entered a new era of all-round development and will make more contributions to the health and well-being of the people of the world in the future.

# Section 2
## Producing Area, Collection, and Storage of Chinese Medicinals

Except for a few artificial products, such as Rengong Niuhuang (Bovis Calculus Artifactus) and Rengong Shexiang (Moschus Artifactus), the vast majority of Chinese medicinals come from the animals, plants, or minerals in nature. They are either hidden in forests, fields, rock caves, or found in the deep sea. Since different types of Chinese medicinals grow in different environments, which significantly affect the efficacy of medicinals, we call those medicinal materials from preferable places of origin with good quality "genuine regional medicines". Coming from the production of Chinese medicinals and the clinical practice of traditional Chinese doctors, and proved by countless TCM clinical practices over thousands of years, it is a standard for distinguishing the quality of Chinese crude medicines from ancient times. Genuine regional medicines often have better efficacy, and modern studies have confirmed that their effective components are significantly higher than those of similar Chinese medicinals.

Different Chinese crude medicines have their unique picking seasons and storage methods. According to the types of medicines and the medication parts, we can divide them into the following categories:

Whole herb: Whole herbs are often picked in the season when plants grow and develop most vigorously, such as in spring and summer. For those medicines that contain roots for medicinal purposes, we should uproot the whole plant when picking. At the same time, attention should be paid to protecting the roots and not exerting excessive force, so as not to damage the plants and affect the efficacy of Chinese medicinals. We should also pay attention to the temperature and humidity in the storage of whole herbs, and the storage area should be large, so as not to cause an excessive backlog of the Chinese medicinals and damage the whole herbs.

Flower, pollen, leaf, and root: In terms of flowers and leaves, we should also pay attention to the picking season. For example, when flowers are harvested, we should pick flower buds that have not yet opened or flowers that have just opened. At this time, the Chinese crude medicine has the best efficacy. Pollens should be collected when flowers are in full bloom, so that we can obtain most medicines. In terms of leaves, we should pay attention to picking them when the plants are in full foliage, so that the leaves contain the most effective ingredients in this period. When collecting roots, we should use the gentle picking technique to avoid any damage to the roots. In terms of the storage of flowers, leaves, and roots of Chinese medicinals, humidity should be kept under control, otherwise they will be stale.

Bark and root bark: Summer is the most suitable season for picking bark medicines. In this season, plants thrive, so the whole plant has sufficient sap content and contains more effective components. Meanwhile, collecting barks can also reduce plant damage to the lowest extent. For root barks, the picking season should be autumn, when the root growth state is the best. Care should be taken to avoid insect bites during storage.

Animal medicine: Most insect medicines, such as Tubiechong (Eupolyphaga Steleophaga), Banmao (Mylabris), Quanxie (Scorpio), Dilong (Pheretima), Lougu (Gryllotalpa), etc., should be captured in late summer and early autumn. During this period, the temperature and the humidity are higher, which is suitable for the growth of insects and is the best season for capture. Sangpiaoxiao (Mantidis Oötheca) is the egg sheath of mantis, and Fengfang (Vespae Nidus) is the hive of wasp. These medicines are mainly collected after the egg sheath and hive formation in autumn. Some animal medicines, such as Shetui (Serpentis Periostracum), is the skin shed by many types of snakes, including black-tail snakes. Since it does not harm the animals, these medicines can be harvested as long as snakes molt. Insect medicines often become fragile when dried in the shade, so attention should be paid to avoid excessive damage during storage.

Mineral medicine: Its composition is relatively stable and can be collected all year round, regardless of time. Store in a cool and ventilated place.

# Section 3
## Processing of Chinese Medicinals

The processing methods of Chinese medicinals include preparation (purifying, crushing, cutting medicinal materials), water processing (rinsing, soaking, moistening, spraying, levigating), fire processing (dry-frying, stir-frying, calcining, roasting), water-fire co-processing (boiling, steaming, stewing, quenching), and other processing methods (frosting, fermenting, germinating, refining, mixing). The purpose of processing Chinese medicinals can be summarized as reducing toxicity and increasing efficacy. For example, boiling Caowu (Aconiti Kusnezoffii Radix) and Chuanwu (Aconiti Radix) with Gancao (Glycyrrhizae Radix et Rhizoma) water and boiling Gansui (Kansui Radix) with vinegar can have the effect of reducing toxicity; while processing Dahuang (Rhei Radix et Rhizoma) with wine and stir-frying Mahuang (Ephedrae Herba) with honey can increase efficacy. In addition, the processing is also a process of sorting pure medicinal materials and distinguishing the grades of medicines. Whether it is a Chinese crude medicine with a lot of sediment or a valuable medicinal material that needs to be priced according to grades, such as Dongchongxiacao (Cordyceps) and Lurong (Cervi Cornu Pantotrichum), the sorting of medicinal materials is an important work before they go into the market. In terms of medicine treatment, drying, slicing, and flavor modifying are the critical steps in processing Chinese medicinals.

# Section 4
## Concerted Application of Chinese Medicinals

The most prominent characteristic of TCM in treating diseases is the concerted application of many Chinese medicinals, which eventually results in the decoctions composed of many kinds of medicinals we are familiar with. Mr. Zhu Shenyu, a late famous doctor in the Peking Union Medical College Hospital, often said that "using medicinals is like commanding soldiers". If each medicine is regarded as a soldier, how to match between the arms and how to grasp their proportion has become the knowledge of military use. Using medicinal also faces the same problem.

In hundreds of Chinese medicinals, how do you know whether the concerted application of different medicinals increases or decreases the efficacy? Is it less toxic or more toxic? During thousands of years of medical practice, our ancients observed the possible results caused by the combined use of different medicinals for a long time and summarized the application of single medicine and the compatibility relationship between medicinals into seven aspects, which were called the "seven relations" of Chinese medicinals, recorded in *Shennong's Classic of Materia Medica*, the earliest extant book of Chinese materia medica in China. The "seven relations" include medicinal used singly, mutual reinforcement, mutual assistance, mutual restraint, mutual suppression, mutual inhibition, and mutual antagonism, the latter six of which vividly describe the relationship between the two medicinals used in combination. The principles of concerted application of medicinals in our TCM prescriptions today are mainly obtained from here.

The so-called **medicinal used singly** refers to the treatment with a single medicinal, which is suitable for a relatively simple disease, so we can select a medicinal with strong pertinence, such as using Huangqin (Scutellariae Radix) alone to treat mild cough with lung heat.

**Mutual reinforcement** refers to the combination of medicinals with similar properties and efficacy enhancing their original curative effect. For example, sometimes, many constipated patients cannot get better even after taking Dahuang (Rhei Radix et Rhizoma). Still, by adding Yuanming Powder, immediate results can be achieved.

**Mutual enhancement** refers to the combined application of medicinals with some common properties and efficacy, with one as the main medicinal and the other as the auxiliary medicinal to improve the curative effect of the former. For example, when heat-fire clearing Huangqin (Scutellariae Radix) is combined with Dahuang (Rhei Radix et Rhizoma) that promotes catharsis and purges heat, Dahuang (Rhei Radix et Rhizoma) can improve the curative effect of clearing heat-fire of Huangqin (Scutellariae Radix).

**Mutual restraint and mutual suppression** means that the concerted application can reduce the toxic side effects of one of the medicinals. For example, the toxicity of unprocessed Banxia (Pinelliae Rhizoma) and unprocessed Tiannanxing (Arisaematis Rhizoma) can be alleviated and eliminated by Shengjiang (Zingiberis Rhizoma Recens), so we can say that unprocessed Banxia (Pinelliae Rhizoma) and unprocessed Tiannanxing (Arisaematis Rhizoma) are incompatible with Shengjiang (Zingiberis Rhizoma Recens), and we can also say that Shengjiang (Zingiberis Rhizoma Recens) counteracts the toxicity of unprocessed Banxia (Pinelliae Rhizoma) and unprocessed Tiannanxing (Arisaematis Rhizoma).

**Mutual inhibition** refers to the combination of two medicinals, in which one medicinal acts with the other and leads to the reduction of the original efficacy or even the loss of efficacy. For example, Renshen (Ginseng Radix et Rhizoma) is inhibited by Laifuzi (Raphani Semen). It is generally believed that Laifuzi (Raphani Semen) can weaken the qi-invigorating effect of Renshen (Ginseng Radix et Rhizoma).

**Mutual antagonism** refers to the combination of two medicinals producing toxic reactions or side effects, such as several concerted applications of medicinals in the "eighteen antagonisms" and the "nineteen mutual inhibitions" in Chinese materia medica.

Among the "seven relations", there are only two kinds of unreasonable concerted applications: mutual inhibition and mutual antagonism. When treating diseases with compound prescriptions of Chinese medicinals clinically, especially in the process of home diet therapy, we should pay more attention to learning the concerted application, not only to make the medicine suitable for our constitution and syndrome, but also to learn the reasonable matching between food ingredients and medicinal materials, so as to achieve the goal of increasing efficacy and reducing toxicity.

# Section 5
## Contraindications of Chinese Medicinals

Although Chinese medicinals are relatively safe and effective, we should also pay attention to their contraindications in daily life and clinical medication, which mainly include contraindications of concerted application, contraindications of choosing medicinals for syndromes, dietetic contraindications, contraindications during pregnancy, etc.

Contraindications of concerted application mainly consist of "eighteen antagonisms" and "nineteen mutual inhibitions" recognized by TCM during medication. The so-called "Rhymed Formula of Eighteen Antagonisms" was first seen in *Confucians' Duties to Parents* by Zhang Zihe of the Jin Dynasty, which refers to: Aconite (including Caowu, Aconiti Kusnezoffii Radix; Chuanwu, Aconiti Radix, and Fuzi, Aconiti Lateralis Radix Praeparata) clashes with Banxia (Pinelliae Rhizoma), Trichosanthes (Gualou, Trichosanthis Fructus; Gualoupi, Trichosanthis Pericarpium; Gualouzi, Trichosanthis Semen; Tianhuafen, Trichosanthis Radix), Fritillaria (such as Zhebeimu, Fritillariae Thunbergii Bulbus; Chuanbeimu, Fritillariae Cirrhosae Bulbus; Pingbeimu, Fritillariae Ussuriensis Bulbus, etc.), Bailian (Ampelopsis Radix), and Baiji (Bletillae Rhizoma); Gancao (Glycyrrhizae Radix et Rhizoma) clashes with Haizao (Sargassum), Daji (Euphorbiae Pekinensis Radix), Yuanhua (Genkwa Flos), and Gansui (Kansui Radix); Lilu (Veratri Radix et Rhizoma) clashes with Ginseng medicines (such as Renshen, Ginseng Radix et Rhizoma; Dangshen, Codonopsis Radix; Xiyangshen, Panacis Quinquefolii Radix; Danshen, Salviae Miltiorrhizae Radix et Rhizoma; Xuanshen, Scrophulariae Radix; Kushen, Sophorae Flavescentis Radix; Nanshashen, Adenophorae Radix; and Beishashen, Glehniae Radix), Xixin (Asari Radix et Rhizoma), Baishao (Paeoniae Radix Alba), and Chishao (Paeoniae Radix Rubra). "Rhymed Formula of Nineteen Mutual Inhibitions" was first seen in *Shallow Reading of Medical Classics* by Liu Chun of the Ming Dynasty, which refers to: Liuhuang (Sulfur) incompatible with Mangxiao (Natrii Sulfas), Shuiyin (Mercury) incompatible with Pishuang (White Arsenic), Langdu (Euphorbiae Ebracteolatae Radix) incompatible with Mituoseng (Litharge), Badou (Crotonis Fructus) incompatible with Qianniuzi (Pharbitidis Semen), Dingxiang (Caryophylli Flos) incompatible with Yujin (Curcumae Radix), Mangxiao (Natrii Sulfas) incompatible with Sanleng (Sparganii Rhizoma), Chuanwu (Aconiti Radix) and Caowu (Aconiti

Kusnezoffii Radix) incompatible with Xijiao (Rhino Horn), Renshen (Ginseng Radix et Rhizoma) incompatible with Wulingzhi (Trogopteri Faeces) and Rougui (Cinnamomi Cortex) incompatible with Chishizhi (Halloysitum Rubrum).

The contraindications of choosing medicinals for syndromes mainly concern that medicinals are tendentious. From the perspective of yin and yang, there are cold and hot medicinals; from the standpoint of ascending and descending, there are medicinals that tend to ascend or descend; from the view of reinforcing and reducing, there are medicinals that tend to tonify or purge. The core of the application of Chinese medicinals is to correct the human body's tendency. If the clinical diagnosis and treatment are improper and the application is wrong, i.e., the medicinal fails to correspond with the syndrome, it may aggravate the illness.

The so-called dietetic contraindications are contraindications on certain foods while taking Chinese medicinals. For example, cold, raw, greasy, and irritating foods should be routinely avoided. It is generally believed by TCM that cold and raw foods inhibit the growth of yang qi in the human body and distress stomach yang, greasy foods are easy to produce phlegm, resulting in the accumulation of pathological products, and irritating foods are likely to consume qi and stir blood. These three kinds of foods will affect the rehabilitation process of diseases to a certain extent and prolong the illness time.

The main contraindications during pregnancy imply that some Chinese medicinals have the side effects of damaging fetal primordial qi and inducing miscarriage. Therefore, for pregnant women, daily and clinical medications unfavorable to the mother, fetus, and labor should be prohibited, including toxic Chinese medicinals (such as Qianniuzi, Pharbitidis Semen; Xionghuang, Realgar; Chuanwu, Aconiti Radix; Maqianzi, Strychni Semen; and Zhuyazao, Gleditsiae Fructus Abnormalis) and those with smooth property or strong power of promoting blood circulation for removing blood stasis and activating qi flowing (such as Taoren, Persicae Semen; Honghua, Carthami Flos; Dahuang, Rhei Radix et Rhizoma; Rougui, Cinnamomi Cortex; and Qumai, Dianthi Herba).

# Section 6

## Dosage, Preparation, and Usage of Chinese Medicinals

The dosage of Chinese medicinals refers to the general dosage adopted by clinicians. Although Chinese medicinals are relatively safe, with an extensive range of safe dosages, and the dosage is not as strict as Western medicine, the clinical efficacy is greatly affected by the dosage. If the dosage is too small, the therapeutic effect will not be achieved, but if the dosage of medicinals is too large, it will also damage the healthy qi of the human body and cause the waste of medicinal resources. Therefore, a reasonable choice of dosage is the key to the application practice of Chinese medicinals. For the usage of Chinese medicinal preparations, generally speaking, the dosage of similar medicinals in pills and powders is less than that in decoctions. Besides, in a prescription, the dosage of the sovereign medicinal that provides the main therapeutic effect is larger than that of complementary medicinals.

The usage of Chinese medicinals mainly concerns the administration route, decoction method, and medication method. Chinese medicinals have a wide range of administration routes, which, in addition to conventional oral administration and external use (skin administration), also include sublingual, rectal, and mucosal administration, etc. With the development of modern pharmaceutical technology, there derive many administration routes, such as intramuscular, subcutaneous, intravenous, and acupoint injection. The main decoction method of Chinese medicinals is soaking the medicinal pieces to be decocted for 30 to 90 minutes, so as to give full play to the efficacy of Chinese medicinals during decocting, and the water surface is generally higher than the surface of medicinal pieces. The decoction is usually done two times. The first time is a conventional decoction, while the water volume added at the second time is about 1/2 of the first decoction. After removing the residue and mixing the two decoctions, the medicine should be taken twice, once in the morning and once in the evening. The grasp of decocting temperature and time should depend on the specific properties of medicinals. Generally speaking, superficies-relieving and heat-clearing medicinals should be decocted quickly on high heat, with the decocting time strictly controlled. After boiling, they can be decocted for 3 to 5 minutes. Otherwise, it will reduce the efficacy of the medicinals. Supplementing Chinese medicinals should be simmered over low heat and then decocted for 30 to 60 minutes after boiling, so that the effective ingredients can be fully released. The conventional way of taking Chinese medicinals is generally one dose daily, to be taken twice a day. The medicine is generally taken warm and should be taken at least 30 minutes apart from diet, to avoid the digestion and absorption of food affecting the efficacy of Chinese medicinals. In addition, according to the lesion sites, the medication methods are also different. For example, as for the diseases above the chest diaphragm, such as headache, dizziness, eye diseases, nasal congestion, and sore throat, medicine should be taken after meals; as for the diseases below the chest diaphragm, such as spleen, stomach, liver, kidney and other viscera diseases, medicine should be taken before meals. Since taking Chinese medicinals before meals can give full play to the efficacy and facilitate the digestion and absorption of medicines, most medicines should be taken before meals. Still, in some cases, such as for certain Chinese medicinals that irritate the gastrointestinal tract, they should be taken after meals.

# Section 7

## Application of Chinese Medicinals

## I Understanding of "toxicity" of Chinese medicinals

Ancient and modern doctors have different opinions on whether Chinese medicinals are "toxic". However, based on the original thinking of TCM, considering the toxicity of Chinese medicinals from a macro perspective, we can regard this toxicity as the tendency of Chinese medicinals in treating diseases. Zhang Jingyue, a famous doctor in Ming Dynasty, said in *Classified Canon*: "Medicinals can cure diseases because of toxicity, and the so-called toxicity is due to the tendency of their qi and flavors. Those with right qi and flavor belong to grains and foods and are used to maintain people's vital qi. Those with tendentious qi and flavor belong to medicines and are therefore used to remove people's pathogenic qi. When people are sick, the disease is due to the tendency of yin or yang... Any medicinal that can drive away pathogenic qi and settle vital qi can be called toxic medicine, so it is said that toxic medicinal attacks pathogens." It is precisely because of the tendency of Chinese medicinals that it can adjust the tendency of the human body, which can be summarized as "correcting tendency by tendency". From this point of view, the concept of "toxicity" in Chinese materia medica mainly reflects its idea of tendency, while the real sense of this word is what we call hepatic and renal toxicity or other visceral toxicity in today's concept. Currently, China has carried out strict control over the use of toxic Chinese medicinals. China's State Council has issued the "Administrative Measures for the Control of Toxic Medicines for Medical Use", which points out that toxic Chinese medicinals include arsenolite, white arsenic, mercury, unprocessed Maqianzi (Strychni Semen), unprocessed Chuanwu (Aconiti Radix), unprocessed Caowu (Aconiti Kusnezoffii Radix), unprocessed Baifuzi (Typhonii Rhizoma), unprocessed Fuzi (Aconiti Lateralis Radix), unprocessed Banxia (Pinelliae Rhizoma), unprocessed Tiannanxing (Arisaematis Rhizoma), unprocessed Badou (Crotonis Fructus), Banmao (Mylabris), Qingniangchong (Lytta Caraganae), Hongniangchong (Huechys Sanguinea), unprocessed Gansui (Kansui Radix), unprocessed Langdu (Euphorbiae Ebracteolatae Radix), unprocessed Tenghuang (Gamboge), unprocessed Qianjinzi (Euphorbiae Semen), unprocessed Tianxianzi (Hyoscyami Semen), Naoyanghua (Rhododendri Mollis Flos), Xueshangyizhihao (Aconiti Brachypodi Radix), Hongsheng Pill, Baijiang Pill, Chansu (Bufonis Venenum),

Yangjinhua (Daturae Flos), Hongfen (Hydrargyri Oxydum Rubrum), Qingfen (Calomelas), and Xionghuang (Realgar). Therefore, we should distinguish the concepts of toxicity and tendency instead of confusing them.

## II  Chinese medicinals and medicine-food homology

China has a long history of homologous medicine and food. Many classics of Chinese medicinals have recorded contents related to food therapy and care of Chinese medicinals. The homologous substances of medicine and food themselves can be used as practical Chinese medicinal materials, and also have the function of diet and are widely used in the field of medical care. Some Chinese medicinals with relatively mild properties and weak tendencies can become important sources of health-preserving food products. For example, Baihe (Lilii Bulbus), Bohe (Menthae Herba), Gouqizi (Lycii Fructus), Juhua (Chrysanthemi Flos), Ejiao (Asini Corii Colla), Shanyao (Dioscoreae Rhizoma), Yiyiren (Coicis Semen), Meiguihua (Rosae Rugosae Flos), Fengmi (Mel), Heye (Nelumbinis Folium), Heizhima (Sesami Semen Nigrum), Machixian (Portulacae Herba), Pugongying (Taraxaci Herba), Lianzi (Nelumbinis Semen), Ganjiang (Zingiberis Rhizoma), and Dazao (Jujubae Fructus) are all materials of medicine-food homology commonly seen in our life. TCM not only focuses on the nutrition of food, but also pays more attention to the nature and flavor of food. TCM theory holds that medicinals have four qi of cold, heat, warmth and coolness, and five flavors of pungent, sweet, acid, bitter and salty. At the same time, medicinals have their own attributed meridians and collaterals, and food is no exception. Therefore, they must be applied with syndrome differentiation based on the constitution of cold, heat, excess or deficiency. According to the nature of the food, for the treatment of heat syndrome, cold food is mostly used; while food for treatment of cold syndrome mostly has warm or hot nature. The efficacy of food can be determined according to five flavors: acid flavor has the effect of astringing, bitter flavor has the effect of descending and purging, sweet flavor has the effect of tonifying, pungent flavor has the effect of scattering, salty flavor has the effect of softening. Acid foods usually have the effects of astringing, promoting fluid production and arresting diarrhea. Bitter foods mostly have the effects of clearing heat, purging fire and detoxifying. Sweet foods usually have the effects of nourishing and moistening intestines. Pungent foods usually have the effects of relieving the surface and promoting qi circulation. Salty foods usually have the effects of softening hardness, dispersing accumulation, and removing blood stasis. Therefore, TCM practitioners also apply diet therapy based on syndrome differention according to the relationship between five flavors and attributed meridians of food and their efficacies. The general rule is: pungent entering the lung, sweet entering the spleen, acid entering the liver, bitter entering the heart, and salty entering the kidney.

# Section 8

## Differences between Chinese Medicinals and Western Medicines

Chinese medicinals have complex components, and each medicine contains several chemical ingredients. The ancients often understood Chinese medicinals based on philosophical thinking, and their application of it also came from experience rather than experiment, so the efficacy of Chinese medicinals is holistic. Unlike Chinese medicinals, Western medicines are based on chemical ingredient theory, with relatively single components and apparent pharmacological effects. However, when we treat Chinese medicinals and Western medicines correctly from the perspective of TCM thinking, they often lead to the same destination in clinical diagnosis and treatment. Western medicine believes that a significant cause of diseases is cell mutation, either the hypofunction or hyperfunction of cells. For those with cell hypofunction, TCM often uses Chinese medicinals that benefit vital qi to invigorate qi, enrich blood, nourish yin and cultivate yang. For those with cell hyperfunction, Chinese medicinals that eliminate pathogenic factors and detoxify are often used to eradicate pathological products that should not exist in the human body, such as phlegm and blood stasis, so as to regulate the balance of body-spirit unity, the balance of qi movement, and the balance of yin and yang. Therefore, we should not only dialectically look at the differences between Chinese medicinals and Western medicines, but also diverge our thinking and cognitive methods and try our best to find the similarities between them to guide clinical practice better.

# Section 9

## The Position of Chinese Medicinals in the National Healthcare System

### The interpretation of Chinese policies related to Chinese medicinals

On July 1, 2017, the Law of the People's Republic of China on Traditional Chinese Medicine (hereinafter referred to as the TCM Law) was officially implemented. TCM Law is the first programmatic, standard and fundamental law in the field of TCM, and is of great significance to standardizing the diagnosis and treatment of TCM in china. It also, for the first time, clarified the important position, development policy, and support measures of TCM from the perspective of national law, which provided a tangible legal guarantee for the development of TCM and laid a legal foundation for the future development of TCM industry in China. With 9 chapters and 63 articles in total, the TCM Law covers many aspects related to the development of TCM, including general provisions, TCM services, protection and development of TCM, training of TCM talents, scientific research of TCM, inheritance and cultural dissemination of TCM, safeguard measures, and legal responsibilities. The national policy normative document most related to Chinese medicinals is *Pharmacopoeia of the People's Republic of China* (hereinafter referred to as *Chinese Pharmacopoeia*), which is the most critical component of Chinese medicine standard and also a code that must be followed in the process of developing, producing, managing, applying, and supervising new medicines. Every five years, Chinese Pharmacopoeia Commission organizes experts to compile a new edition of *Chinese Pharmacopoeia* and appropriately updates the existing content based on the latest clinical research. The current edition is the 2020 edition of *Chinese Pharmacopoeia*, with a total of four parts, of which the first part mainly records Chinese medicinals, the second part contains chemicals, the third includes biological products, and the fourth embodies general technical requirements and pharmaceutic excipients. The fact that *Chinese Pharmacopoeia* puts Chinese medicinals at the core of the first part, which also clarifies the important position of Chinese medicinals in the field of medicine application in China. In addition, in recent years, China has continuously issued documents that benefit the Chinese materia medica industry. For example, in January 2021, the General Office of the State Council published "Several Policies and Measures on Accelerating the Characteristic Development of Traditional Chinese Medicine", which clearly states the necessity to improve the vitality of the Chinese materia medica industry and enhance the vigor of TCM development. The publication of such documents greatly focuses on the dilemma and difficulties in developing TCM, which reflects the support and investment of China's policy in TCM.

## II  The policies of other countries around the world on Chinese medicinals

The Dietary Supplement Health and Education Act, enacted in 1994, is a federal law of the USA that not only defines dietary supplements but also provides for safety and efficacy claims. Its definition of "dietary supplement" includes "herbs or other plants" and "any concentrate" thereof, which confirms the legal status of plant extracts as dietary supplements.

Germany has a certain system for the management of Chinese medicinals, such as allowing plant extracts to be registered as prescription medicines in the legislative procedure, which, to some extent, affirms the role of Chinese medicinals. About 60,000 registered medicines in Germany contain herbal ingredients, most of which are herbal extracts. These medicines are based on 600–700 plants, and about 5,000 kinds of extracts or preparations have been produced. Nevertheless, Germany also is very strict in the examination and approval of Chinese medicinals. For example, if a Chinese medicinal wants to enter Germany as a botanical medicine, there will be complicated approval procedures. Only when the contents of pesticides, heavy metals, and microorganisms do not exceed the standard and their quality meets certain requirements, can they enter the German market for sale. Currently, most Chinese medicinals enter Germany as healthcare products and are applied according to the procedure of food management.

Although Japan has been deeply influenced by Chinese culture throughout history and is the largest export market of Chinese medicinals, the use of Hanfang medicine is also greatly restricted. Currently, except for the approved 210 kinds of prescriptions, the Ministry of Health, Labour and Welfare of Janpan is stringent in the approval of new Hanfang Medicine, treating them in the same way as new compound medicines. Moreover, there are many restrictive measures for the approval of imported traditional Chinese patent medicines. But in recent years, the Japanese government has significantly eased its control over healthy food, such as canceling the restrictions on dosage forms and relaxing the restrictions on the types of natural plant medicines that can be used in healthy food. Japan has introduced the new Pharmaceutical Law, the basic principle of which is "deregulation". The management measures for medicine production and circulation are getting increasingly closer to those in Europe and the United States. The previous strict restrictions will be relaxed.

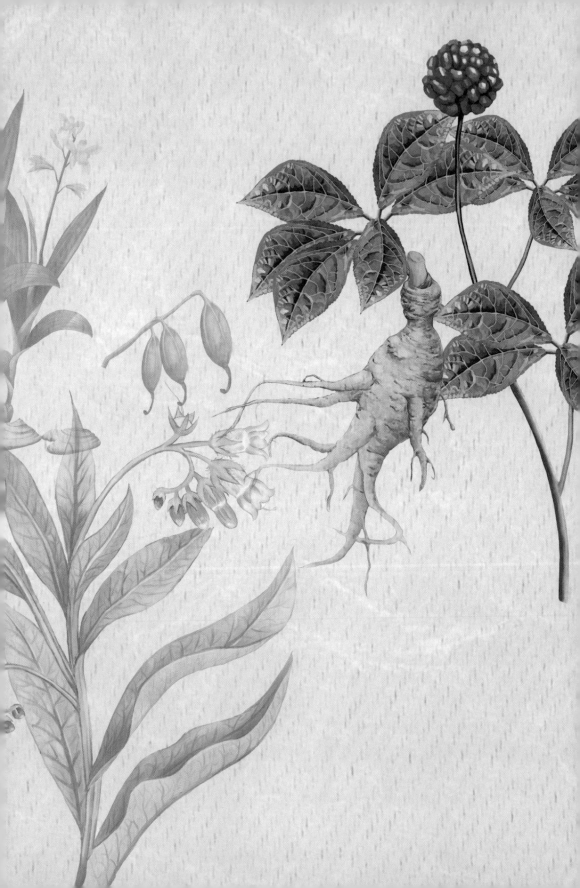

Chapter 2

Guidelines for the Commonly

Used Chinese Medicinals

# Section 1
## Chinese Medicinals Used for Both Medicine and Food

### I  Baihe (Lilii Bulbus)

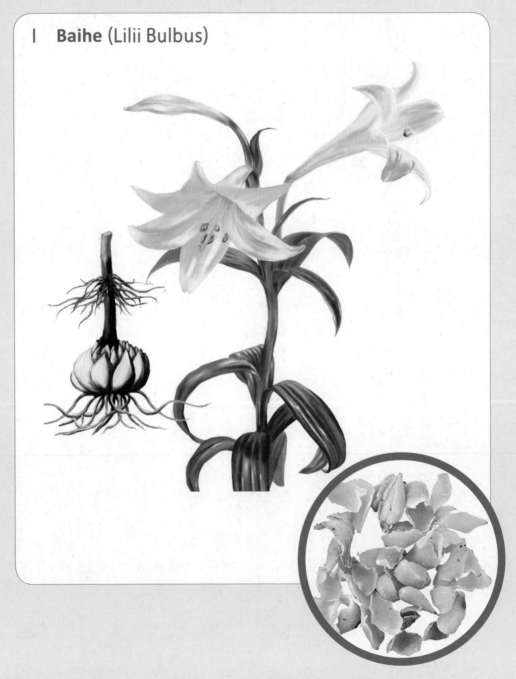

◎ *Which part of the plant is used as Baihe (Lilii Bulbus)?*

The bulbs of Liliaceae plants such as *Lilium lancifolium* Thunb., *Lilium brownii* F. E. Brown var. *viridulum* Baker, or *Lilium pumilum* DC.

◎ *Where is the best Baihe (Lilii Bulbus) produced?*

Baihe (Lilii Bulbus) produced in Hunan is regarded as good quality.

◎ *How to distinguish the quality of Baihe (Lilii Bulbus)?*

It is better to have uniform and thick petals, yellow and white appearance, firm quality, fewer tendons, and a bitter taste.

◎ *How to preserve Baihe (Lilii Bulbus)?*

Baihe (Lilii Bulbus) should be stored in a warm place instead of a cold one, and it is not resistant to wind. After being exposed to the wind, it is easy to turn red and wither. Rinse fresh Baihe (Lilii Bulbus) with clear water to remove mucus, dry it in the sun or in a heater. If you want to use it fresh, you can bury Baihe (Lilii Bulbus) in fine sand for storage, and the storage temperature should be 5–11 °C; the dried Baihe (Lilii Bulbus) can be stored in a dry and cool place.

◎ *What is the difference between raw Baihe (Lilii Bulbus) and the honey-fried?*

Baihe (Lilii Bulbus) decoction pieces are divided into raw Baihe (Lilii Bulbus) and honey-fried Baihe (Lilii Bulbus). The former has a good effect of clearing heart fire and calming the mind, while the latter has a good effect of nourishing yin and moistening the lung.


[Efficacy Told by the Doctor]


◎ *Medicinal properties and efficacy—nourishing yin, moistening the lung, and clearing the heart*

Baihe (Lilii Bulbus) tastes sweet, and is slightly cold. It enters the lung and heart meridians and has a tonic effect. Its color is white; TCM believes that white color mainly enter the lung, so it can nourish yin and moisten the lung. In addition, it also has a certain cough expectorant effect, and external use can treat skin carbuncle and eczema.

◎ *Applicable people—yin deficiency constitution, dry throat, chronic cough, dysphoria, and insomnia*

Baihe (Lilii Bulbus) is mainly suitable for people with yin deficiency and internal heat in the heart, lung, and stomach, and is mostly used for those who are thin, cannot bear heat, prone to night sweats, have dry mouth, and want to drink cold water, and have dry stool, less and yellow urine.

Patients with yin deficiency and lung dryness mainly present dry cough with less phlegm, hemoptysis, dry throat, hoarseness, dysphoria and vexing heat, night sweat, and so on.

Patients with deficiency heat disturbing the heart may present insomnia, palpitation, trance, uncontrollable emotion, bitter taste, yellow urine, and so on.

Patients with yin deficiency and stomach heat mainly present dry mouth and lips, gastric upset, retching, decreased food intake, discomfort in chest and diaphragm after eating, dry stool, and so on.

◎ *Applicable syndrome*

Baihe (Lilii Bulbus) can be used for the treatment of patients with yin deficiency and lung dryness, deficiency heat disturbing the heart and yin deficiency and stomach heat manifested by pulmonary tuberculosis and high fever in convalescent period, neurosis, menopausal syndrome, advanced lung cancer, chronic gastritis, duodenal ulcer and advanced gastric cancer.

◎ *What kinds of people are not suitable for Baihe (Lilii Bulbus)?*

Because Baihe (Lilii Bulbus) is slightly cold and has the function of nourishing yin and astringing lung, it is not suitable for people who cough with exogenous wind-cold, usually cannot bear the cold but like warmth, have a cold stomach and like to drink warm water, with loose stool.

If one cannot bear the cold, have a cold stomach, and diarrhea after taking Baihe (Lilii Bulbus), he/she should stop using it, and take gingerade appropriately to relieve symptoms.

## [Diet Therapy Recommended by the Doctor]

◎ *Usage and dosage of Baihe (Lilii Bulbus) in diet therapy*

Baihe (Lilii Bulbus) is sweet and gentle in medicinal property, and 5–15g can be used as a substitute for tea in daily life. For home meals such as stir-frying, cooking soup, porridge, etc., 10 –30g can be used for decoction pieces and 30–60g for fresh Baihe (Lilii Bulbus).

◎ *What season is Baihe (Lilii Bulbus) most suitable for taking?*

Baihe (Lilii Bulbus) can be taken all year round because it has the function of nourishing yin and clearing heart fire. It is especially suitable for taking in summer and autumn.

◎ *How to combine Baihe (Lilii Bulbus) with other medicinal materials and food ingredients?*

Baihe (Lilii Bulbus) is sweet, cold, and moist. For the effects of nourishing yin, especially nourishing lung yin, it is often accompanied by white sugar or Fengmi (Mel) to enhance its yin-nourishing and dryness-moistening effects. It is often combined with Shengdihuang (Rehmannia Radix), Yuzhu (Polygonati Odorati Rhiozma), Maidong (Ophiopogonis Radix), Chuanbeimu (Fritillariae Cirrhosae Bulbus), Zhebeimu (Fritillariae Thunbergii Bulbus), etc., for the treatment of deficiency of lung yin, manifested by dry cough with less sputum or blood in sputum, vexing heat in the palms and soles, night sweat, etc.

In daily cooking, it is often matched with celery, bitter gourd, bamboo shoots, and other heat-clearing and urination-promoting ingredients to play the role of clearing heat and nourishing yin; it can often be matched with mung beans, Yiyiren (Coicis Semen), etc., to be cooked as congee to clear heat and strengthen the spleen; it can often be matched with black-bone chicken, Yuzhu (Polygonati Odorati Rhiozma) and Gouqizi (Lycii Fructus) to be cooked as soup to nourish yin and moisten dryness.

◎ *How to choose Baihe (Lilii Bulbus) and Yuzhu (Polygonati Odorati Rhiozma) in diet therapy?*

Baihe (Lilii Bulbus) and Yuzhu (Polygonati Odorati Rhiozma) are sweet and cold, which have the therapeutic effects of clearing lung heat, nourishing yin, clearing heat and promoting fluid production. They are often used together to improve the curative effect of each other. Compared with Yuzhu (Polygonati Odorati Rhiozma), Baihe (Lilii Bulbus) can clear the heart heat and tranquillize the mind. Therefore, it is more suitable to choose Baihe (Lilii Bulbus) in case of dysphoria, insomnia, palpitation, and dreaminess.

**Small experiential recipe**

*1. To treat chronic belching and abdominal distension repeatedly*
Fresh Baihe (Lilii Bulbus) 30g, Wuyao (Linderae Radix) 9g. Both medicinals are cooked as soup, and taken warm, once in the morning and once in the afternoon.

*2. To treat insomnia and neurasthenia*
Fresh Baihe (Lilii Bulbus) 60g is mixed with an appropriate amount of Fengmi (Mel) and then steamed, and taken before going to bed.

*3. To treat unhealed ulcer wound*
Fresh Baihe (Lilii Bulbus) 100g, together with a little borneol is mashed, mixed well and applied to the affected area, once a day.

## ‖ **Bohe** (Menthae Herba)

◎ *Which part of the plant is used as Bohe (Menthae Herba)?*

The dry aerial part of Labiatae plant *Mentha haplocalyx* Briq..

◎ *Where is the best Bohe (Menthae Herba) produced?*

Suzhou area, Jiangsu Province has large output and high quality.

◎ *How to distinguish the quality of Bohe (Menthae Herba)?*

It is better to have many leaves, dark green color, cool taste, and strong aroma. It is generally believed that the cultivated herb in Taicang, Jiangsu Province has the best quality.

◎ *How to preserve Bohe (Menthae Herba)?*

Fresh Bohe (Menthae Herba) is usually dried in the sun or dried in the shade after cutting. Keep dried Bohe (Menthae Herba) in a cool place.

◎ *What is the difference between leaves and stalks?*

Bohe (Menthae Herba) leaves have better sweating and exterior-relieving effects, while Bohe (Menthae Herba) stalks tend to circulate qi and harmonize the middle.

[Efficacy Told by the Doctor]

◎ *Medicinal properties and efficacy—dispersing wind-heat, refreshing dizziness and blurred vision, relieving sore throat and promoting eruption, dispersing stagnated liver qi for relieving qi stagnation*

Bohe (Menthae Herba) is cool and pungent: pungent flavor is to disperse, and cool property is to clear heat. It belongs to the lung meridian and has the function of dispersing wind and heat. Its color is green, and TCM believes that green color mainly enters the liver meridian, and its nature is pungent and dispersing, so it can disperse stagnated liver qi to relieve qi stagnation. In addition, it also has a certain effect of eliminating foul qi and can be used to treat vomiting and diarrhea due to summer-heat-dampness.

◎ *Applicable people—exogenous wind-heat, headache, red eyes, chest tightness, and hypochondriac pain*

Bohe (Menthae Herba) is mainly suitable for people with the exogenous wind-heat pathogen and is mostly used for people with a strong constitution who catch a cold due to wind-heat, manifested as fever, slight aversion to wind-cold, dry throat, thirst, headache, and red eyes.

Bohe (Menthae Herba) can disperse stagnated liver qi and promote qi circulation, and treat people with a stagnation of liver qi, manifested as chest and hypochondriac pain and menstrual disorders.

◎ *Applicable syndrome*

Bohe (Menthae Herba) can be used to treat wind-heat cold, headache, sore throat, sores in mouth and tongue, rubella, measles, chest and abdomen distension, tightness, etc. In addition, Bohe (Menthae Herba) also has anti-inflammatory and analgesic effects.

◎ *What kinds of people are not suitable for Bohe (Menthae Herba)?*

Because Bohe (Menthae Herba) is cold, fragrant and pungent, and it will make people sweat and consume qi, so it is not suitable for people with physical deficiency and hyperhidrosis, spleen deficiency and loose stool. Pregnant women, women giving birth, and young children should avoid eating it.

Toxic and side effects of Bohe (Menthae Herba) are rare. Taking Bohe (Menthae Herba) oil by mistake may cause dizziness, blurred vision, nausea, vomiting, numbness of hands and feet, gradual coma, and a slight drop in blood pressure.

**[Diet Therapy Recommended by the Doctor]**

◎ *Usage and dosage of Bohe (Menthae Herba) in diet therapy*

Bohe (Menthae Herba) have a special cool fragrance, which can disperse wind and heat, clear the head and eyes, relieve sore throat, promote eruption, and disperse stagnated liver qi for relieving qi stagnation. 5–15g can be used as a substitute for tea in daily life. For home meals such as cake, soup, and porridge, 15g can be used for decoction pieces and 30g for fresh Bohe (Menthae Herba). However, Bohe (Menthae Herba) contains aromatic volatile oil, it is better to cover it when making tea, and the time for making tea or decocting soup should not be too long, generally 5–6 minutes.

◎ *What season is the most suitable for us to take Bohe (Menthae Herba)?*

Bohe (Menthae Herba) can be taken all year round, and it is especially suitable for taking in spring and summer because of its effects of dispelling wind and heat, eliminating filth and turbidity.

◎ *How to combine Bohe (Menthae Herba) th other medicinal materials and food ingredients?*

Bohe (Menthae Herba) is pungent and cool, and it is more compatible with Jinyinhua (Lonicerae Japonicae Flos), Lianqiao (Forsythiae Fructus), Niubangzi (Arctii Fructus), Jingjie (Schizonepetae Herba), etc.,for dispersing wind-heat. If it is used for the stagnation of liver qi and stuffy pain in the chest and hypochondrium, it is often combined with Chaihu (Bupleuri Radix), Baishao (Paeoniae Radix Alba), and Danggui (Angelicae Sinensis Radix).

Bohe (Menthae Herba) can be combined with mung beans and Yiyiren (Coicis Semen) to clear heat and strengthen the spleen when cooking porridge; when making cakes, it is used with mung beans and glutinous rice to clear heat and wind; when cooking, it can be combined with tofu and shredded chicken to clear heat.

**Small experiential recipe**

*1. To treat cough and sore throat caused by lung heat*
Bohe (Menthae Herba) 10g, olives 50g, radish 100g. Put the above three ingredients into a pot, add water to decoct them, and take the medicinal juice.

*2. To treat tinnitus and deafness caused by phlegm-qi block*
Dried tangerine peel 10g, reed rhizome 10g, water chestnuts 3 pieces, Bohe (Menthae Herba) 6g. Wash the above materials except for Bohe (Menthae Herba) and put them into a pot, add water to boil the soup, finally add Bohe (Menthae Herba) and boil it slightly, then turn off the fire, and take the juice as tea.

# Ⅲ **Gouqizi** (Lycii Fructus)

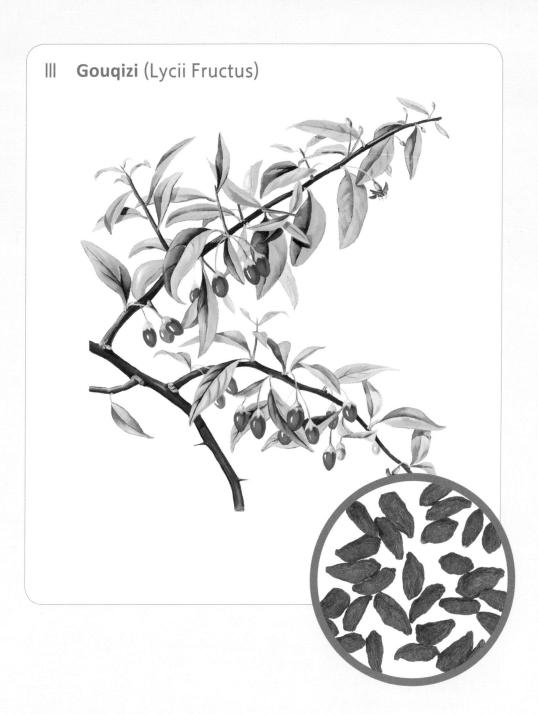

◎ *Where is the best Gouqizi (Lycii Fructus) produced?*

Gouqizi (Lycii Fructus) produced in Ningxia, Gansu, and Qinghai is regarded as good quality.

◎ *How to distinguish the quality of Gouqizi (Lycii Fructus)?*

It is better to have large fruits, red color, thick flesh, few seeds, soft and moist texture, and sweet taste.

◎ *How to preserve Gouqizi (Lycii Fructus)?*

Gouqizi (Lycii Fructus) contains much sugar, which is easy to absorb moisture and oil, prone to be moldy, or moth-eaten, and it is easy to change color. It is a simple and practical method to store at 0–4°C in a refrigerator.

[Efficacy Told by the Doctor]

◎ *Medicinal properties and efficacy—nourishing the kidney, enriching the liver, improving eyesight, and moistening the lung*

Gouqizi (Lycii Fructus) tastes sweet and its nature is not biased, has a tonifying effect, and is good at nourishing yin of the liver and kidney. TCM believes that eyes are the window of the liver, and the eye essence belongs to the kidney; while the liver and kidney yin are sufficient, the eyes are bright, so Gouqizi (Lycii Fructus) can improve eyesight. By nourishing yin of the liver and kidney, it has the function of nourishing blood and can treat sallow complexion. It can promote fluid production and quench thirst, and at the same time, it enters the lung meridian to nourish yin and moisten the lung.

◎ *Applicable people—yin deficiency constitution, dry throat, chronic cough, dysphoria, and insomnia*

Gouqizi (Lycii Fructus) is placid, without obvious bias, and its effectiveness is moderate, without hindering digestion. People with weak constitutions can take it frequently for a long time. It is mainly suitable for people with yin essence insufficiency of the liver and kidney and deficiency of yin and blood and is mostly used for people with a thin body, dark yellow complexion, sore waist, weak legs, insomnia and dreaminess, prematurely white hair and beard, and loose teeth.

Those with yin deficiency of the liver and kidney and inability to control yang often present dizziness, soreness of the waist and legs, blurred vision, and so on.

Those with liver and kidney deficiency and depletion of yin and blood often present insomnia, dreaminess, and sallow complexion.

Those who are mainly injured by internal heat often have dry mouth and lips, gastric upset, retching, decreased diet, discomfort in chest and diaphragm after eating, dry stool, and so on.

◎ *Applicable syndrome*

Gouqizi (Lycii Fructus) can be used for the treatment of anemia, chronic fatigue syndrome, chemical liver injury, diabetes, hyperlipidemia, hypertension, tumor, chronic atrophic gastritis, infertility, etc., which belong to the syndromes of liver and kidney deficiency and depletion of yin and blood.

◎ *What kinds of people are not suitable for Gouqizi (Lycii Fructus)?*

Gouqizi (Lycii Fructus) is less greasy, but it is sweet and moist after all. Therefore, those who have weak spleen and stomach, and loose stools, cannot bear the cold and like warmth, and those who like to drink warm water with a cold stomach should use less Gouqizi (Lycii Fructus).

[Diet Therapy Recommended by the Doctor]

◎ *Usage and dosage of Gouqizi (Lycii Fructus) in diet therapy*

Gouqizi (Lycii Fructus) is sweet and placid in medicinal properties, and

5–10g can be used as a substitute for tea in daily life. For home meals such as stir-frying, cooking soup, porridge, etc., 5–15g of decoction pieces and 10–30g of fresh Gouqizi (Lycii Fructus) can be used.

◎ *What season is Gouqizi (Lycii Fructus) most suitable for taking?*

Gouqizi (Lycii Fructus) can be taken all year round because it has the function of nourishing the liver and kidney, especially suitable for taking in autumn and winter.

◎ *How to combine Gouqizi (Lycii Fructus) with other medicinal materials and food ingredients?*

Gouqizi (Lycii Fructus) is sweet and its nature is not biased, and when it is used to nourish the liver and kidney, especially to nourish the liver and improve eyesight, it is often added with Shudihuang (Rehmanniae Radix Praeparata) and Juhua (Chrysanthemi Flos) to enhance the effects; for the treatment of deficiency of yin and blood and sallow complexion, it can be boiled with eggs, and can also be boiled with Longyanrou (Longan Arillus) for those with insomnia and dreaminess.

In daily porridge cooking, it is often combined with ingredients such as Shanyao (Dioscoreae Rhizoma) and glutinous rice to invigorate qi and spleen; when making soup, it can often be combined with black-bone chicken, Yuzhu (Polygonati Odorati Rhizoma), and Baihe (Lilii Bulbus) to nourish yin and moisten dryness.

◎ *How to choose Gouqizi (Lycii Fructus) and Sangshen (Mori Fructus) as a diet therapy?*

Sangshen (Mori Fructus) is sweet and cold and has the effects of nourishing yin and enriching blood, promoting fluid production, and moistening intestines. They can be used together to enhance the effects of nourishing the liver and kidney and benefiting yin and blood. At the same time, Sangshen (Mori Fructus) can moisten intestines better than Gouqizi (Lycii Fructus), so it is more suitable to choose Sangshen (Mori Fructus) for patients with blood deficiency, intestinal dryness, constipation, internal heat, and thirst.

*1. To treat Infertility*

Chew 15g of Gouqizi (Lycii Fructus) every night, and take it for one month as a course of treatment.

*2. To treat chronic atrophic gastritis*

Gouqizi (Lycii Fructus) 20g per day, take it twice a day on an empty stomach, and 2 months is a course of treatment.

*3. To treat dizziness, fainting, and tinnitus*

30–60g of Gouqizi (Lycii Fructus) is decocted in water every day, and take it frequently.

# IV  **Jinyinhua** (Lonicerae Japonicae Flos)

## [Drug Selection by the Pharmacist]

◎ *How many kinds of Jinyinhua (Lonicerae Japonicae Flos) are there? Which is better?*

Jinyinhua (Lonicerae Japonicae Flos) is divided into Mi Yinhua and Ji Yinhua according to the producing areas, and Mi Yinhua produced in Henan is regarded to have a better quality.

◎ *How to distinguish the quality of Jinyinhua (Lonicerae Japonicae Flos)?*

The flower buds newly opened, complete, yellow and white in color and free of impurities are  characteristics of good quality.

◎ *How to preserve Jinyinhua (Lonicerae Japonicae Flos)?*

The fresh medicinal should be firstly dried in a cool place, and then stored in a dry and ventilated place.

◎ *What is the difference among raw flower, charred flower and distillate?*

Jinyinhua (Lonicerae Japonicae Flos) can be used in the form of raw, charred, and distillate. Raw Jinyinhua (Lonicerae Japonicae Flos) disperses wind and heat, and especially has a good effect of clearing heat in the interior. Charred Jinyinhua (Lonicerae Japonicae Flos) has lost the function of clearing heat, but the effects of cooling blood, detoxifying and stopping dysentery are good. Jinyinhua distillate has the effect of clearing heat and relieving summer heat.

## [Efficacy Told by the Doctor]

◎ *Medicinal properties and efficacy—clearing heat and detoxifying, dispersing wind-heat, cooling blood and stopping dysentery*

TCM believes that Jinyinhua (Lonicerae Japonicae Flos) has light weight, and has the function of evacuating wind and heat. With sweet and cold properties, it belongs to the lung, heart and stomach meridians, and can clear away heat and detoxify. Its smell is fragrant, and it can also relieve the poison in the blood.

◎ *Applicable people—lung heat constitution, sore throat, sores, carbuncles, furuncles, heat toxin and diarrhea*

Jinyinhua (Lonicerae Japonicae Flos) is mainly suitable for people with lung heat constitution. It is mostly used for cold tolerance, exogenous wind-heat, sore throat, fever, sweating, thirst, sores, carbuncles, swelling and toxin, and dysentery with pus and blood.

Patients contracted with wind-heat mainly present fever, headache, sore throat and thirst.

Patients with sores, carbuncles and furuncles mainly present local redness, swelling, heat and pain, pus and even ulceration.

Patients with heat toxin diarrhea mainly present diarrhea with pus and blood, borborygmus and abdominal pain, fecal difficulty, burning anus and so on.

◎ *Applicable syndrome*

Jinyinhua (Lonicerae Japonicae Flos) can be used for treating febrile diseases with fever, heat toxin and bloody dysentery, carbuncle, swelling, furuncle and various infectious diseases.

◎ *What kinds of people are not suitable for Jinyinhua (Lonicerae Japonicae Flos)?*

Because Jinyinhua (Lonicerae Japonicae Flos) is cold in nature, those with weak constitution, loss of appetite, cold intolerance and preference for warmth, loose stool, and spleen and stomach deficiency cold should take it with caution. People with insufficient healthy qi, clear pus discharge after sores are ruptured are not suitable for taking it.

If there is fear of cold, cold stomach and loose stool after taking Jinyinhua (Lonicerae Japonicae Flos), stop using it, and take Rougui (Cinnamomi Cortex) appropriately to relieve the symptoms.

◎ *Usage and dosage of Jinyinhua (Lonicerae Japonicae Flos) in diet therapy*

Jinyinhua (Lonicerae Japonicae Flos) is sweet and cold, and 5–10g can be used as a substitute for tea in daily life.

◎ *What season is Jinyinhua (Lonicerae Japonicae Flos) best for taking?*

Jinyinhua (Lonicerae Japonicae Flos) can be taken all year round. Because it has the functions of clearing away heat and detoxifying, it is especially suitable for taking in summer.

◎ *How to combine Jinyinhua (Lonicerae Japonicae Flos) with other medicinal materials and food ingredients?*

Jinyinhua (Lonicerae Japonicae Flos) is sweet, cold and light, and is often combined with Jingjie (Schizonepetae Herba), Bohe (Menthae Herba) and Lianqiao (Forsythiae Fructus) to dispel exterior pathogen and treat common cold due to wind-heat pathogens. For those with sores, carbuncles and furuncles, it is often combined with Pugongying (Taraxaci Herba), Yejuhua (Chrysanthemi Indici Flos) and Huangqin (Scutellariae Radix). For treating dysentery with blood and pus due to heat toxin, it can be combined with Huanglian (Coptidis Rhizoma), Huangqin (Scutellariae Radix) and Baitouweng (Pulsatillae Radix) to enhance the effects of clearing heat, cooling blood and stopping dysentery.

It can be matched with japonica rice to make Jinyinhua (Lonicerae Japonicae Flos) porridge to clear away heat and relieve summer heat. Herbal tea made with Heye (Nelumbinis Folium) and Jinyinhua (Lonicerae Japonicae Flos) can prevent heatstroke, cold and intestinal infectious diseases.

◎ *How to choose Jinyinhua (Lonicerae Japonicae Flos) and Rendongteng (Lonicerae Japonicae Caulis) as a diet therapy?*

Jinyinhua (Lonicerae Japonicae Flos) and Rendongteng (Lonicerae Japonicae Caulis) have similar functions, both of which have diet therapy effects such as clearing heat, detoxifying and dispersing wind-heat. However, Rendongteng

(Lonicerae Japonicae Caulis) is not as effective as Jinyinhua (Lonicerae Japonicae Flos) in dispersing wind-heat exterior pathogen, but it has the effects of dredging collaterals and relieving pain. Oral administration is for the treatment of joint redness, heat pain, unfavorable flexion and extension, etc.

### Small experiential recipe

*1. To treat heat toxin and sores*

Rendongteng (Lonicerae Japonicae Caulis), Huangqi (Astragali Radix) and Gancao (Glycyrrhizae Radix et Rhizoma) are cut into thin pieces in a ratio of 2 : 4 : 1, soaked in wine, decocted and taken.

*2. To treat dysentery due to heat toxin*

100–200g of Rendongteng (Lonicerae Japonicae Caulis), decocted in water and taken.

# V  **Juhua** (Chrysanthemi Flos)

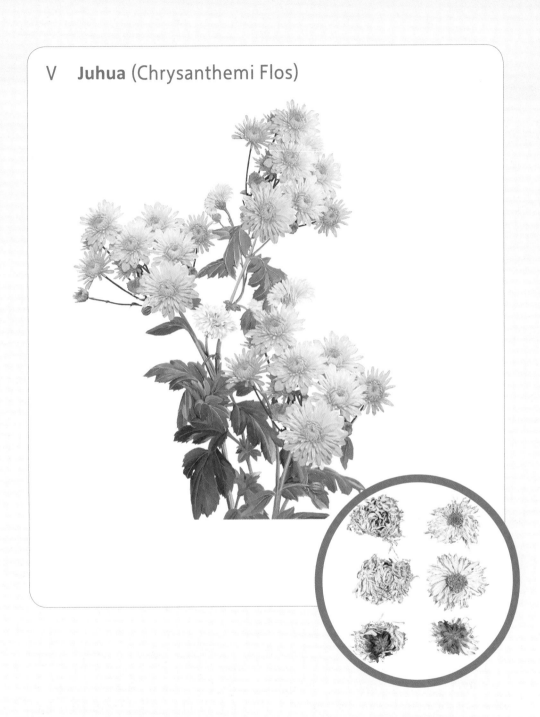

◎ *Where is the best Juhua (Chrysanthemi Flos) produced?*

Boju (Chrysanthemi Flos) produced in Bozhou of Anhui Province, and Shangqiu of Henan Province, and Chuju (Chrysanthemi Flos) produced in Chuzhou of Anhui Province are regarded as good quality.

◎ *How to distinguish the quality of Juhua (Chrysanthemi Flos)?*

Juhua (Chrysanthemi Flos) is better with dry, white (yellow), and complete flowers, rich aroma, and no impurities.

◎ *How to preserve Juhua (Chrysanthemi Flos)?*

It should be stored in a cool and dry place to avoid humidity.

◎ *What is the difference between yellow Juhua (Chrysanthemi Flos) and white Juhua (Chrysanthemi Flos)?*

Yellow Juhua (Chrysanthemi Flos) (commonly known as Hangju) is used to scatter wind and heat, and white Juhua (Chrysanthemi Flos) (commonly known as Chuju) is used to calm the liver and improve eyesight.

◎ *Medicinal properties and efficacy—dispelling wind, calming the liver, clearing heat, and improving eyesight*

Juhua (Chrysanthemi Flos) is pungent and light in texture. TCM believes that pungent medicinals can disperse qi and blood, reach the head and face, and reach the muscle surface outside, so it can dispel wind. Its nature is slightly cold, and TCM believes that medicinals with cold nature can clear heat, so it can dispel wind and clear heat. It enters the lung meridian and can treat fever, sore throat, cough and other symptoms caused by wind-heat invading the lung. In addition, it also enters the liver meridian, which can disperse wind-heat and stabilize liver yang, thus treating headache and dizziness caused by hyperactivity of liver yang. It can also clear liver fire, improve eyesight and relieve nebula to treat red eyes, swelling, and pain caused by inflammation of liver fire.

◎ *Applicable people—damp-heat constitution, wind-heat invading the lung, hyperactivity of liver yang, and inflammation of liver fire*

Juhua (Chrysanthemi Flos) is mainly suitable for people with the damp-heat constitution, and mostly used for those who are impatient, fearful of heat, prone to fever, have sore throat and sweating after catching a cold, and want to drink cold water with a dry mouth, dry stool, and yellow urine.

Due to wind-heat invading the lung, after catching a cold, patients tend to have a severe fever, slight aversion to wind, head pain, redness and pain in the throat, cough, sticky or yellow sputum, stuffy nose, yellow nasal discharge, thirst with a desire to drink.

Patients with hyperactivity of liver yang are irritable, dizzy, and have headaches.

Patients with liver fire flaming upward have red eyes, swelling, pain, facial furuncle, and so on.

◎ *Applicable syndrome*

Juhua (Chrysanthemi Flos) can be used for the treatment of colds, fever, pharyngitis, hypertension, conjunctivitis, and other diseases due to wind-heat invading the lung, hyperactivity of liver yang, and liver fire flaming upward.

◎ *What kinds of people are not suitable for Juhua (Chrysanthemi Flos)?*

Because Juhua (Chrysanthemi Flos) is slightly cold, it is not suitable for people with cough, headache and aversion to cold due to externally contracted wind-cold, fear of cold and liking warmth, a cold stomach and liking to drink warm water, and thin stool.

If one cannot bear the cold, has a cold stomach, and diarrhea after taking Juhua (Chrysanthemi Flos), he/she should stop using it, and take gingerade appropriately to relieve the symptoms.

◎ *Usage and dosage of Juhua (Chrysanthemi Flos) in diet therapy*

Juhua (Chrysanthemi Flos) is slightly cold and gentle in medicinal properties, so it is best to take 3—5g as tea in daily life.

◎ *What season is Juhua (Chrysanthemi Flos) most suitable for taking?*

Juhua (Chrysanthemi Flos) can be taken all year round. Because it has the function of dispelling wind and clearing heat, it is especially suitable for taking in spring and summer.

◎ *How to combine Juhua (Chrysanthemi Flos) with other medicinal materials and food ingredients?*

For wind-dispelling and heat-clearing effects, it is often boiled with Bohe (Menthae Herba), Jinyinhua (Lonicerae Japonicae Flos), Sangye (Mori Folium), etc., to drink as tea; for the effect of stabilizing liver yang, it is often boiled with Tianma (Gastrodiae Rhizoma) and Gouteng (Uncariae Ramulus cum Uncis) to drink as tea; for the effects of clearing the liver, purging heat and improving eyesight, it is boiled with Juemingzi (Cassiae Semen), Gouqizi (Lycii Fructus), Xiakucao (Prunellae Spica), Gujingcao (Eriocauli Flos), etc., to drink as tea.

◎ *How to choose Juhua (Chrysanthemi Flos) and Yejuhua (Chrysanthemi Indici Flos) as a diet therapy?*

Juhua (Chrysanthemi Flos) and Yejuhua (Chrysanthemi Indici Flos) are both pungent and slightly cold with the effects of dispelling wind and clearing heat. They are often used together to improve the curative effect of each other. However, Yejuhua (Chrysanthemi Indici Flos) is more powerful in clearing heat and detoxifying, and more suitable for facial furuncle or boil.

## Small experiential recipe

*1. To treat cold, fever, dizziness, red eyes, and throat discomfort*

Juhua (Chrysanthemi Flos) 6g, Bohe (Menthae Herba) 9g, Jinyinhua (Lonicerae Japonicae Flos) 10g, and Sangye (Mori Folium) 10g are boiled for drinking as tea.

*2. To prevent and treat early hypertension*

10g of Juhua (Chrysanthemi Flos) and 3g of tea are boiled for drinking as tea.

*3. To treat red eyes and dizziness due to liver heat*

Juhua (Chrysanthemi Flos) 10g, dry-fried Juemingzi (Cassiae Semen) 12g. Boil them for drinking as tea.

# VI Ejiao (Asini Corii Colla)

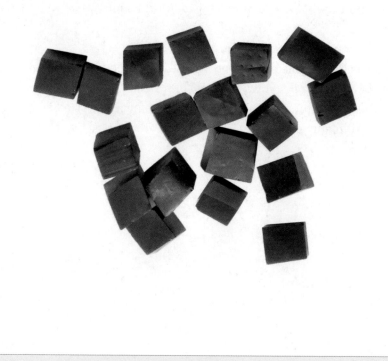

**[Drug Selection by the Pharmacist]**

◎ *How to distinguish the authenticity of Ejiao (Asini Corii Colla)?*

Ejiao (Asini Corii Colla) should be as yellow as amber and as black as paint. True Ejiao (Asini Corii Colla) has no skin odor, and is not wet or soft in summer. When holding the gelatin with hand and flapping it on the tabletop, if the cross-section of the fragment is brown, translucent, and free of foreign body, it is true; if it is soft but not broken, it is proved to be fake.

◎ *How to preserve Ejiao (Asini Corii Colla)?*

Ejiao (Asini Corii Colla) is easy to dry and break when exposed to wind for a long time, become soft when exposed to the sun, and easy to regain moisture and soften if affected by dampness and heat. The safe moisture content is 16%–18%. If the moisture content exceeds 21%, mold will grow. If the relative humidity is below 75%, the moisture will be lost and the gelatin will be brittle. Therefore, the suitable relative humidity for storage is 80%–85%. If too much moisture is absorbed, it can be dried with burnt lime and lime chloride. When the summer air is hot and humid, it should be stored in the refrigerator.

◎ *What are the differences among Ejiao (Asini Corii Colla), Guijiajiao (Testudinis Carapacis et Plastri Colla) and Lujiaojiao (Cervi Cornus Colla)?*

As for Guijiajiao (Testudinis Carapacis et Plastri Colla), its surface is brown and slightly green, with a yellow "oily texture" on it, which is as clean as amber and hard in quality; as for Lujiaojiao (Cervi Cornus Colla), its surface is black-brown, and it is translucent with yellow-white porous thin layer on one side, brittle, and red-brown in transverse section, with glass luster.

### [Efficacy Told by the Doctor]

◎ *Medicinal properties and efficacy — enriching blood, nourishing yin, moistening the lung, and stopping bleeding*

Ejiao (Asini Corii Colla) tastes sweet, and TCM believes that sweet medicinal has a tonic effect. Ejiao (Asini Corii Colla) is animal product and therefore is vital for enriching blood. It is believed that Ejiao (Asini Corii Colla) can enter the lung, liver, and kidney meridians to nourish yin and blood, so this medicine also has the functions of nourishing yin, moistening the lung and nourishing the liver and kidney. In addition, it is sticky in quality and can be used to stop bleeding.

◎ *Applicable people — people with deficiency of both yin and blood, hemorrhagic disease*

Ejiao (Asini Corii Colla) is mainly suitable for people with deficiency of both yin and blood, especially for patients with deficiency of both yin and blood of the lung, liver, and kidney. It is mostly used for spitting blood and nosebleeds due to yin deficiency and blood heat, metrorrhagia and metrostaxis due to blood deficiency and deficiency cold, palpitation, cough with less phlegm, dry throat, blood-stained sputum, vexation, and sleeplessness.

Patients with lung heat and yin deficiency present cough with less phlegm, dry throat, and blood-stained sputum.

People with kidney yin deficiency and hyperactivity of heart fire present vexation and sleeplessness.

◎ *Applicable syndrome*

Ejiao (Asini Corii Colla) is good at treating various diseases caused by blood deficiency, and plays a role in moistening the skin by enriching blood, regulating menstruation, protecting the fetus, strengthening the physique, improving sleep, promoting brain development and improving brain function, delaying aging. It can also be used for the treatment of neurasthenia, dizziness, insomnia, dreaminess, fatigue, and other diseases.

◎ *What kinds of people are not suitable for Ejiao (Asini Corii Colla)?*

Because Ejiao (Asini Corii Colla) is sweet and sticky, it should be used with caution for those with weak spleen and stomach, vomiting and diarrhea, abdominal distension and loose stool, cough, and excessive phlegm. It is not suitable for cold patients. Pregnant women, children and patients with hypertension and diabetes should take it under the guidance of a doctor. Women during menstruation should use it with caution or under the guidance of a doctor. People with yin deficiency and yang hyperactivity need to reduce the amount or frequency as appropriate to prevent excessive internal heat symptoms such as sore throat. The specific symptoms of yin deficiency and yang hyperactivity are as follows: dry mouth in the morning, many eye droppings, dry stool, and irritability.

**[Diet Therapy Recommended by the Doctor]**

◎ *Usage and dosage of Ejiao (Asini Corii Colla) in diet therapy*

Ejiao (Asini Corii Colla) can be completely melted and refrigerated, and taken with warm boiled water every day. 5–10g can be used for home dishes such as soup and porridge.

◎ *What season is Ejiao (Asini Corii Colla) most suitable for taking?*

Ejiao (Asini Corii Colla) can be taken all year round. In late winter and early spring, the whole body begins to flourish just like plants, so this is the best time to eat tonic food. Taking Ejiao (Asini Corii Colla) at this time can often play a very good role in uplifting yang qi.

◎ *How to combine Ejiao (Asini Corii Colla) with other medicinal materials and food ingredients?*

Ejiao (Asini Corii Colla) is sweet and neutral in nature. Because it has the function of enriching blood and stopping bleeding, it's better to treat blood deficiency caused by bleeding. For this, it is often combined with Shudihuang (Rehmanniae Radix Praeparata), Danggui (Angelicae Sinensis Radix), Baishao (Paeoniae Radix Alba), etc.; to treat cough due to lung yin deficiency, it is often combined with Niubangzi (Arctii Fructus) and Kuxingren (Semen Armeniacae Amarum).

When cooking it for porridge, it can be combined with rock sugar to enrich blood and tonify the kidney; pear, rock sugar, eggs, or other ingredients can be added to make soup to moisten the lung and stop coughing.

---

**Small experiential recipe**

*To treat cough due to lung dryness and excessive phlegm due to long-term illness*
Ejiao pear Fengmi (Mel) soup: Cut one or two pears into small pieces; add some water, and boil them; add Ejiao (Asini Corii Colla) 12g (smashed), stir repeatedly with chopsticks to dissolve; add 50g of white sugar or rock sugar and 50g of Fengmi (Mel). Eat the pear with soup.

# VII Shanyao (Dioscoreae Rhizoma)

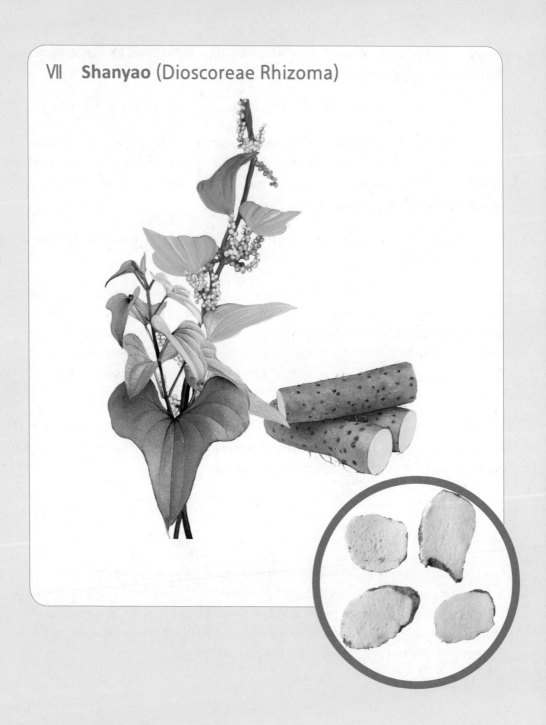

## [Drug Selection by the Pharmacist]

◎ *Which part of the plant is used as Shanyao (Dioscoreae Rhizoma)?*

The rhizome of Dioscoreaceae plant *Dioscorea opposita* Thunb. is used as Shanyao (Dioscoreae Rhizoma), raw or fried with bran.

◎ *Where is the best Shanyao (Dioscoreae Rhizoma) produced?*

Shanyao (Dioscoreae Rhizoma) produced in Huaiqing, Henan Province is regarded as good quality, so it is called "Huai Shanyao".

◎ *How to distinguish the quality of Shanyao (Dioscoreae Rhizoma)?*

It is better to have a large tuber with mucous flesh (mucus can be seen when it is broken), more root hair, no damage to the outer skin, white transverse section, and low moisture content.

◎ *How to preserve Shanyao (Dioscoreae Rhizoma)?*

Shanyao (Dioscoreae Rhizoma) is cold-resistant and can be stored locally when necessary. The suitable storage temperature is 0–2°C, and the relative humidity is about 90%. The common storage method is the basket storage: the sun-sterilized straw or wheat straw is laid around the sterilized basket or box. Then pile the selected Shanyao (Dioscoreae Rhizoma) layer by layer until the basket or box is 80% full, and cover it with wheat straw. Finally, stack it in the warehouse, keep the temperature to prevent moisture on the ground. Bricks or planks can be placed on the bottom of the basket.

◎ *What is the difference between raw product and bran-fried product?*

The decoction pieces of Shanyao (Dioscoreae Rhizoma) are divided into raw Shanyao (Dioscoreae Rhizoma) and bran-fried Shanyao (Dioscoreae Rhizoma). The former has a good effect of tonifying the kidney and consolidating essence, while the latter has a good effect of tonifying the lung and invigorating qi.

◎ *Medicinal properties and efficacy—tonifying the spleen and stomach, promoting fluid production and benefiting the lung, tonifying the kidney, and astringing essence*

Shanyao (Dioscoreae Rhizoma) tastes sweet, has a tonic effect, and enters the lung, spleen, and kidney meridians. Its medicinal properties are not biased, and it can replenish qi and yin, tonify the spleen, lung, and kidney, consolidate essence and stop leukorrhea. Because of its characteristics of supplementing both qi and yin, it also has a certain curative effect on diabetic patients with deficiency of both qi and yin as the main pathogenesis.

◎ *Applicable people—spleen deficiency and excessive dampness, lung deficiency and cough and asthma, kidney deficiency and spermatorrhea*

Shanyao (Dioscoreae Rhizoma) is mainly suitable for people with deficiency of qi and yin in the lung, spleen, and kidney, and is mostly used for people with fatigue, reduced appetite, loose stool, frequent urination at night or enuresis, cough and asthma due to long-term illness, clear and thin leukorrhagia in women, spermatorrhea, night emission and premature ejaculation in men.

Patients with deficiency of spleen qi often present emaciation or obesity, fatigue, reduced appetite, abdominal distension, loose stool, and leukorrhagia in women.

Patients with deficiency of lung qi often present cough, asthma, fatigue, shortness of breath, white and thin expectoration, spontaneous perspiration, aversion to wind, and vulnerability to a cold.

Patients with kidney qi deficiency often present soreness and weakness of the waist and knees, tinnitus and deafness, mental fatigue, weakness, frequent micturition, enuresis, nocturia, spermatorrhea, and premature ejaculation in men, etc.

◎ *Applicable syndrome*

Shanyao (Dioscoreae Rhizoma) can be used for patients with chronic gastritis, chronic nephritis, long-term diarrhea, premature ejaculation, and various chronic diseases due to the above-mentioned pathogenesis such as lung qi deficiency, failure of splenic transportation, and kidney qi deficiency.

◎ *What kinds of people are not suitable for Shanyao (Dioscoreae Rhizoma)?*

Shanyao (Dioscoreae Rhizoma) has the effect of astringency, so it is not suitable for people with dry stool to prevent constipation. In addition, patients who are in the acute stage of nephritis, pneumonia, and other diseases should not eat Shanyao (Dioscoreae Rhizoma).

Shanyao (Dioscoreae Rhizoma) and Gansui (Kansui Radix) should not be eaten together. Nor should it be taken with alkaline drugs.

**[Diet Therapy Recommended by the Doctor]**

◎ *Usage and dosage of Shanyao (Dioscoreae Rhizoma) in diet therapy*

Shanyao (Dioscoreae Rhizoma) is sweet and gentle and is suitable for all kinds of people. According to different cooking methods, such as stir-frying, cooking soup, making porridge, the dosage of home dishes is different. 10–30g can be used for decoction pieces and 30—60g for fresh Shanyao (Dioscoreae Rhizoma).

◎ *What season is Shanyao (Dioscoreae Rhizoma) most suitable for taking?*

Shanyao (Dioscoreae Rhizoma) can be taken all year round, because it has a tonic effect on the lung, spleen, and kidney, and it has its advantages when taken in different seasons. When eaten in autumn it can tonify lung qi; it can strengthen spleen qi when eaten all year round; if taken in winter, it tonifies kidney qi the most.

◎ *How to combine Shanyao (Dioscoreae Rhizoma) with other medicinal materials and food ingredients?*

Shanyao (Dioscoreae Rhizoma) tastes sweet and its medicinal properties are not biased. Combined with Taizishen (Pseudostellariae Radix) and Nanshashen (Adenophorae Radix), it plays the role of tonifying lung qi and relieving asthma. When treating reduced appetite, abdominal distension, and loose stool due to a spleen qi deficiency, it is combined with Dangshen (Codonopsis Radix) and Baizhu (Atractylodis Macrocephalae Rhizoma), and other medicinals to fortify the spleen and boosting qi. When treating kidney deficiency, it is often combined with Dihuang (Rehmannia Radix), Fuling (Poria), and other medicinals to tonify the kidney and promote fluid production. Many famous prescriptions for tonifying the kidney in the past dynasties, such as "Shenqi Pill" and "Liuwei Dihuang Pill", contain Shanyao (Dioscoreae Rhizoma).

In daily cooking, it often goes with black fungus, which not only stimulates appetite but also plays a role in tonifying the kidney. It is often be cooked with Qianshi (Euryales Semen) and Yiyiren (Coicis Semen) as congee to drain dampness and fortify the spleen, and can also be cooked with jujube to supplement qi and blood, strengthen the spleen and stimulate appetite.

◎ *How to choose Shanyao (Dioscoreae Rhizoma) and Qianshi (Euryales Semen) as a diet therapy?*

Shanyao (Dioscoreae Rhizoma) and Qianshi (Euryales Semen) are both sweet and not biased, which have the dietary effects of invigorating the spleen, relieving diarrhea, tonifying the kidney, and consolidating essence. They are often used together to improve the curative effect of each other. Compared with Qianshi (Euryales Semen), Shanyao (Dioscoreae Rhizoma) can also tonify lung qi and nourish lung yin. Therefore, Shanyao (Dioscoreae Rhizoma) is better at treating fatigue, cough, asthma and shortness of breath due to long-term illness.

### Small experiential recipe

*1. To treat weakness of spleen and stomach, reduced appetite and indigestion*

Shanyao (Dioscoreae Rhizoma) 60g, cut into small pieces, Hongzao (Jujubae Fructus) 30g, a proper amount of Jingmi (Oryzae Sativae Semen). The above ingredients are boiled into congee, and seasoned with sugar to eat.

*2. To treat cough and asthma due to long-term illness, with little or no phlegm, dry throat, and dry mouth*

Fresh Shanyao (Dioscoreae Rhizoma) 60g, chopped and mashed; add half a bowl of sugarcane juice, and mix well. Stew the mixture on fire and take it warm.

*3. To treat spermatorrhea, amnesia, insomnia, emaciation, etc.*

Shanyao (Dioscoreae Rhizoma) 50g, Qianshi (Euryales Semen) 50g, Jingmi (Oryzae Sativae Semen) 50g. The above ingrdients are cooked as congee and seasoned with salt. Take it warm every night.

# VIII   Yiyiren (Coicis Semen)

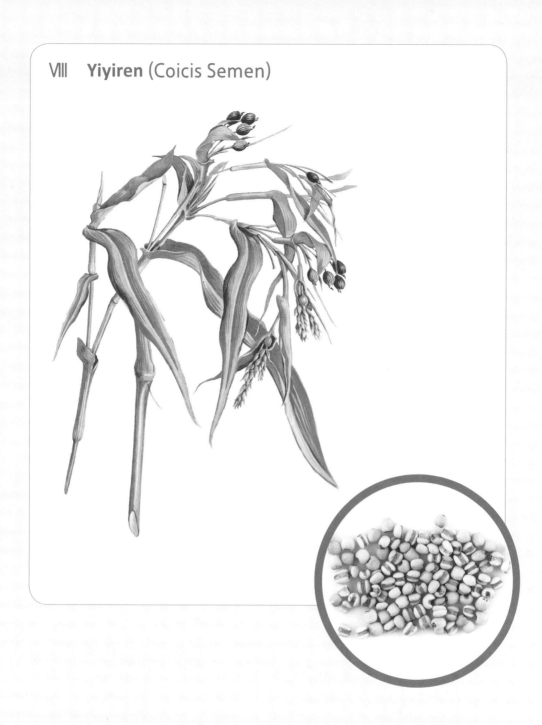

◎ *Which part of the plant is used as Yiyiren (Coicis Semen)?*

The dry ripe kernels of a Gramineae plant *Coix lacryma-jobi* L. var. *ma-yuen* (Roman.) Stapf are used as medicine.

◎ *Where is the best Yiyiren (Coicis Semen) produced?*

Yiyiren (Coicis Semen) is produced in most areas of China, and those produced in Fujian, Hebei and Liaoning are regarded as good quality.

◎ *How to distinguish the quality of Yiyiren (Coicis Semen)?*

High-quality Yiyiren (Coicis Semen) is solid with large and full grains, white color, and unbroken skin.

◎ *How to preserve Yiyiren (Coicis Semen)?*

Yiyiren (Coicis Semen) likes dryness and hates dampness. It should be stored in a ventilated, cool and dry place. The storage temperature should be 5–11°C, and be sure to ward off bugs.

◎ *What is the difference between raw Yiyiren (Coicis Semen) and bran-fried Yiyiren (Coicis Semen)?*

The decoction pieces of Yiyiren (Coicis Semen) are divided into raw Yiyiren (Coicis Semen) and bran-fried Yiyiren (Coicis Semen). The former has a good effect of clearing heat and draining dampness, while the latter has a good effect of invigorating the spleen and arresting diarrhea.

◎ *Medicinal properties and efficacy—clearing dampness, promoting diuresis, strengthening the spleen, clearing heat, expelling pus, and removing arthralgia*

Yiyiren (Coicis Semen) tastes sweet and bland. Its medicinal properties are slightly cool and belong to the spleen, stomach, and lung meridians. It is bland and sweet, which not only promotes diuresis and detumescence, but also strengthens the spleen, invigorates the spleen and stomach and arrests diarrhea, and can also relax muscles, relieve convulsion, clear heat and expel pus. It can treat diarrhea, swelling, dysuria caused by spleen deficiency and excessive dampness, and arthralgia caused by pathogenic wind-damp.

◎ *Applicable people—spleen deficiency and phlegm-dampness constitution, edema, abdominal distension, and arthralgia of muscles and tendons*

Yiyiren (Coicis Semen) is mainly suitable for people with spleen deficiency and excessive dampness constitution, and is mostly used for people with overweight, fatigue, dysuria, diarrhea, and proneness to edema, and also has a certain curative effect on people with cough and spitting thick phlegm due to lung heat.

Patients with spleen deficiency and excessive dampness often present edema, fatigue, sleepiness, thirst and no desire to drink water, abdominal distension, dysuria, and diarrhea.

◎ *Applicable syndrome*

Yiyiren (Coicis Semen) can be used for chronic diarrhea, rheumatoid arthritis, chronic appendicitis, chronic gastritis, heatstroke and beriberi with edema and spleen deficiency diarrhea, and other diseases belonging to spleen deficiency and excessive dampness.

◎ *What kinds of people are not suitable for Yiyiren (Coicis Semen)?*

Yiyiren (Coicis Semen) is suitable for all kinds of people, but because its function is to promote urination and percolate dampness, people with spleen deficiency but with no dampness, dry stool, and no sweat, and pregnant women should take it with caution.

[Diet Therapy Recommended by the Doctors]

◎ *Usage and dosage of Yiyiren (Coicis Semen) in diet therapy*

Yiyiren (Coicis Semen) is easy to take and can be purchased in supermarkets and drugstores. About 60g is appropriate for congee and 150g for soup. It has a slow effect, so it should be taken for a long time and with a considerable amount.

◎ *What season is Yiyiren (Coicis Semen) most suitable for taking?*

Yiyiren (Coicis Semen) can be taken all year round, because of its obvious effects of permeating dampness and promoting diuresis, and it has the best effect when it is taken in summer and long summer (from May to August according to the lunar calendar).

◎ *How to combine Yiyiren (Coicis Semen) with other medicinal materials and food ingredients?*

Yiyiren (Coicis Semen) permeates dampness and promotes diuresis, and is often compatible with Fuling (Poria), Baizhu (Atractylodis Macrocephalae Rhizoma), and Huangqi (Astragali Radix). When treating beriberi edema, it can be used with Fangji (Stephaniae Tetrandrae Radix), Mugua (Chaenomelis Fructus) and Cangzhu (Atractylodis Rhizoma). In addition, it is especially suitable for treating diarrhea due to spleen deficiency and excessive dampness, and is often combined with Renshen (Ginseng Radix et Rhizoma), Fuling (Poria) and Baizhu (Atractylodis Macrocephalae Rhizoma). It is combined with Duhuo (Angelicae Pubescentis Radix), Fangfeng (Saposhnikoviae Radix) and Cangzhu (Atractylodis Rhizoma) for acute pain due to muscle contracture.

When cooking porridge, it can go with Shanyao (Dioscoreae Rhizoma) and mumg beans to clear heat and strengthen the spleen, or be cooked with Jingmi (Semen Oryzae Sativae) to strengthen the spleen to eliminate dampness; when cooking soup, it can also go with mutton to replenish qi and deficiency, strengthen the spleen and kidney.

◎ *How to choose Yiyiren (Coicis Semen) and Fuling (Poria) as a diet therapy?*

Both Yiyiren (Coicis Semen) and Fuling (Poria) can promote diureses to relieve swelling, percolate dampness, and strengthen the spleen. However, Fuling (Poria) is neutral in nature and tonifies the heart and spleen, and calms the heart and tranquillize the mind; Yiyiren (Coicis Semen) is cool and heat-clearing and is good at expelling pus and removing arthralgia. They are often used together and complement each other.

*1. To treat spleen and lung yin deficiency, loss of appetite, deficiency heat, fatigue and cough; chronic belching and abdominal distension repeatedly*

Yiyiren (Coicis Semen) 60g and Shanyao (Dioscoreae Rhizoma) 60g are mashed into coarse powder and boiled in water until well cooked.

*2. To treat damp-heat and blood stasis syndrome, manifested by insomnia, neurasthenia, constipation, short and red urine*

Yiyiren (Coicis Semen) 15g, Dongguazi (Semen Benincasae) 30g, Taoren (Persicae Semen) 10g, Mudanpi (Moutan Cortex) 6g. Decoct them with water and take the decoction.

*3. To treat edema, dysuria, wheezing, and chest fullness*

Yuliren (Pruni Semen) 60g, ground and filtered with water to obtain the liquid; Yiyiren (Coicis Semen) 200g, cooked with the liquid of Yuliren. Take it twice daily.

# IX   Meiguihua (Rosae Rugosae Flos)

◎ *Which family does Meiguihua (Rosae Rugosae Flos) belong to, and what is the medicinal part?*

Meiguihua (Rosae Rugosae Flos) is the flower of the Rosaceae plant, and its medicinal and edible parts are the died buds of a rose.

◎ *Where is Meiguihua (Rosae Rugosae Flos) mainly grown?*

The origin is north China. There are garden cultivations all over China, mainly produced in Jiangsu, Zhejiang, Fujian, Shandong, and Sichuan.

◎ *What are the colors of roses?*

Roses are mainly in red, yellow, purple, white, black, orange, and blue colors. Red and purple roses are the main medicinal and edible ones.

◎ *How to harvest and preserve roses?*

In late spring and early summer, rose buds are picked when they are just open, and the fully expanded but not open buds are picked, dried, or sun dried for later use, or fresh products are also used. Store them in a dry and cool place.

◎ *What is the difference between fresh Meiguihua (Rosae Rugosae Flos) and dried Meiguihua (Rosae Rugosae Flos)?*

Commonly used Meiguihua (Rosae Rugosae Flos) are fresh or dried. The former has a good effect on dispersing stagnated liver qi to relieve qi stagnation, while the latter has a good effect on promoting blood circulation to relieve pain.

[Efficacy Told by the Doctor]

◎ *Medicinal properties and efficacy—dispersing stagnated liver qi to relieve qi stagnation, promoting blood circulation to relieve pain*

Meiguihua (Rosae Rugosae Flos) mainly sweet in taste, slightly bitter in taste, and fragrant in smell has the function of regulating qi and promoting blood circulation and its color is purplish red. TCM believes that it mainly enters the liver meridian and can disperse stagnated liver qi for relieving qi stagnation; it is mild in medicinal property and can promote blood circulation, reduce swelling and relieve pain, and have a good effect of promoting blood circulation to relieve pain. In addition, it has a certain aromatic function of invigorating the spleen and stomach, and can also be used externally to treat traumatic injury, bruise, and pain.

◎ *Applicable people—qi stagnation and blood stasis constitution, depression, and menstrual disorders*

Meiguihua (Rosae Rugosae Flos) is mainly suitable for people with qi stagnation and blood stasis and is mostly used for people with qi stagnation and blood stasis, manifested by a thin body, depression, irregular menstruation, and breast pain.

Patients with stagnation of liver qi mainly have depression, unhappiness, sighing, chest and hypochondriac distension and discomfort.

Patients with blood stasis blocking as the main pathogenesis have heartache, abdominal pain, traumatic injury, swelling and pain, breast distending pain during menstruation, irregular menstruation, dysmenorrhea, dark menstruation with blood clots, etc.

Patients with liver qi invading the stomach have abdominal distension, pain, reduced appetite, nausea, acid regurgitation, and even vomiting.

◎ *Applicable syndrome*

Meiguihua (Rosae Rugosae Flos) can be used to treat depression, hyperplasia of mammary glands, irregular menstruation, dysmenorrhea, stomachache, indigestion, traumatic injury, and other syndromes belonging to qi stagnation and blood stasis.

◎ *What kinds of people are not suitable for Meiguihua (Rosae Rugosae Flos)?*

Meiguihua (Rosae Rugosae Flos) is slightly warm and has the function of promoting qi and blood circulation. Most people are suitable to drink Meiguihua (Rosae Rugosae Flos) tea, especially women. However, because Meiguihua (Rosae Rugosae Flos) can promote blood and circulation, it is advisable to use it less for patients with blood heat and blood deficiency. Patients with bleeding who do not belong to qi stagnation and blood stasis according to TCM syndrome differentiation should not use it.

## [Diet Therapy Recommended by the Doctor]

◎ *Usage and dosage of Meiguihua (Rosae Rugosae Flos) in diet therapy*

Meiguihua (Rosae Rugosae Flos) is fragrant and sweet. 3–6g can be used as tea every day, 10g of fresh Meiguihua (Rosae Rugosae Flos) or 5–10 rose buds can be used.

◎ *What season is most suitable for taking Meiguihua (Rosae Rugosae Flos)?*

Meiguihua (Rosae Rugosae Flos) can be taken all year round because it has the function of dispersing stagnated liver qi to relieve qi stagnation. It is especially suitable for taking in spring.

◎ *How to combine Meiguihua (Rosae Rugosae Flos) with other medicinal materials and food ingredients?*

Meiguihua (Rosae Rugosae Flos) is fragrant, sweet, and warm. When used to treat stagnation of liver qi, manifested as depression, unhappiness, sighing, chest and hypochondrium distension and discomfort, it is often combined with Yuejihua (Rosae Chinensis Flos), Xiangfu (Cyperi Rhizoma), Meihua (Mume Flos), Yujin (Curcumae Radix), Hehuanhua (Albiziae Flos) and Chaihu (Bupleuri Radix) to enhance the effect. It is often combined with Sharen (Amomi Fructus), Shanzha (Crataegi Fructus), Shenqu (Massa Medicata Fermentata), Maiya (Hordei Fructus Germinatus), Xiangyuan (Citri Fructus) and Foshou (Citri Sarcodactylis Fructus) when used to treat liver qi invading the stomach, manifested as abdominal distension and pain in the chest and hypochondrium, eating less food, nausea and acid regurgitation, and even vomiting; when treating blood stasis, manifested as heartache, abdominal pain, traumatic injury, static swelling and pain, breast distension an pain during menstruation, irregular menstruation, dysmenorrhea, dark menstrual blood with clots, etc., it is often used in conjunction with Danshen (Salviae Miltiorrhizae Radix et Rhizoma), Danggui (Angelicae Sinensis Radix), Chuanxiong (Chuanxiong Rhizoma), Sanqi (Notoginseng Radix et Rhizoma), Zelan (Lycopi Herba), Yimucao (Leonuri Herba) and Jiguanhua (Celosiae Cristatae Flos).

In addition, to treat irregular menstruation, Meiguihua (Rosae Rugosae Flos) and rock sugar or brown sugar are boiled to form paste, and stored in porcelain bottles for sealed preservation. One teaspoonful in the morning and 1 teaspoonful in the evening, and taken with warm boiled water. In diet therapy, a proper amount of fresh Meiguihua (Rosae Rugosae Flos) are washed and mashed, and stewed with rock sugar can treat lung disease with hemoptysis or blood in sputum.

◎ *How to choose Meiguihua (Rosae Rugosae Flos) and Yuejihua (Rosae Chinensis Flos) as a diet therapy?*

Both Meiguihua (Rosae Rugosae Flos) and Yuejihua (Rosae Chinensis Flos) can regulate qi, and have the effects of dispersing stagnated liver qi to relieve qi stagnation, promoting qi circulation, and blood flow. They are often used together to improve the curative effect of each other. Compared with Yuejihua (Rosae Chinensis Flos), Meiguihua (Rosae Rugosae Flos) is fragrant and has stronger effects of regulating qi and dispersing stagnated liver qi to relieve qi stagnation. Therefore, it is more suitable for the syndrome of liver qi stagnation, mainly manifested by depression, unhappiness, sighing, chest and hypochondriac distension, and discomfort.

**Small experiential recipe**

*1. To treat stomachache, indigestion, hemoptysis caused by pulmonary disease*
Meiguihua (Rosae Rugosae Flos) 100g is mashed and mixed with white crystal sugar 300g, placed in the sun, and taken after the sugar dissolves. 3 times a day, 10g each time. This paste can be eaten for a long time and has the functions of strengthening the body resistance, harmonizing the spleen and stomach, moistening and beautifying the skin.

*2. To treat globus hystericus with a sensation of a foreign body in the pharynx, which one cannot spit out or swallow.*
Meiguihua (Rosae Rugosae Flos) 12g, Banxia (Pinelliae Rhizoma) 10g, Dazao (Jujubae Fructus) 10g, Zisugeng (Caulis Perillae) 10g. Decocted with water, 1 dose every day.

*3. To treat breast carbuncle and breast swelling pain*
Meiguihua (Rosae Rugosae Flos) 7 pieces, Dingxiang (Caryophylli Fructus) 7 pieces. Decocted with a proper amount of yellow rice wine.

## X  Fengmi (Mel)

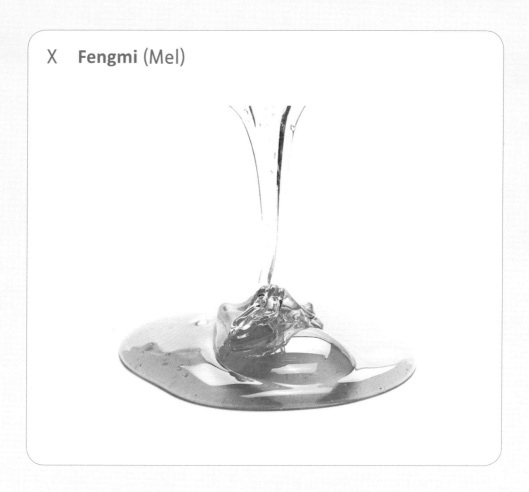

[Drug Selection by the Pharmacist]

◎ *Where is the Fengmi (Mel) produced with better quality?*

It is regarded that Fengmi (Mel) produced in Xinjiang and Hainan is excellent.

◎ *How to distinguish the quality of Fengmi (Mel)?*

According to color, Fengmi (Mel) can be divided into yellow and white, and the ancients took white Fengmi (Mel) as the top. Fengmi (Mel) with clear color, bright luster, stringlike and sticky texture, exquisite crystal, sweet and slightly acid flavor, soft and smoothy taste is characteristic of good quality.

◎ *How to preserve Fengmi (Mel)?*

Fengmi (Mel) is afraid of strong light, because too strong light will greatly destroy the vitamin B group in it, resulting in the loss of nutrients. During the preservation process, Fengmi (Mel) should be placed in a dry, clean, and ventilated environment at low temperature and away from light. The storage temperature should be 5–15°C, and the air humidity should not exceed 75%.

◎ *What is the difference between raw Fengmi (Mel) and boiled Fengmi (Mel)? What other effects does it have?*

Fengmi (Mel) has a cool nature when it is raw, so it can clear heat; when boiled, it becomes warm, so it can invigorate the spleen and stomach. It can detoxify because it is sweet and placid, moisten dryness because it is soft and moist, relieve pain because it is slow and alleviant, and harmonize the medicinal properties and help other medicinals to exert their efficacies.

**[Efficacy Told by the Doctor]**

◎ *Medicinal properties and efficacy—invigorating the spleen and stomach, moistening dryness, relieving pain, detoxifying*

Fengmi (Mel) is sweet, gentle, and slightly warm. It belongs to the spleen, lung, stomach, and large intestine meridians. Sweet taste can enter the spleen, so it can invigorate and strengthen the spleen. When the spleen qi is nourished, food can moisten the intestines. The lung likes to be moist but not dry, while Fengmi (Mel) also enters the lung. Fengmi (Mel) is placid and can relieve pain, harmonize various medicinals and help detoxify at the same time.

◎ *Applicable people—deficiency of spleen and stomach qi, yin deficiency constitution, pain*

Fengmi (Mel) is mainly suitable for people with deficiency of spleen and stomach qi, deficiency of body fluid, and pain. And it is mostly used for people with constipation.

Patients with deficiency of spleen and stomach qi are mainly manifested by poor appetite, poor taste, fatigue, flaccidity, and softness of limbs.

Patients with yin deficiency mainly present tidal fever, night sweats, constipation, dry cough, and hemoptysis.

Patients with pain mainly present by various types of pain due to deficiency of the five internal organs, and muscle pain, sores and ulcers in the heart and abdomen.

◎ *Applicable syndrome*

Fengmi (Mel) can be used to treat stomach pain, constipation, fatigue and pain belonging to yin deficiency or qi deficiency syndrome.

◎ *What kinds of people are not suitable for Fengmi (Mel)?*

The sweet taste tends to be stagnant, so it is forbidden for those with deficiency cold of the spleen and stomach. It is moist and smooth, so it is also forbidden for those with diarrhea. Do not eat Fengmi (Mel) with raw onions. Eating it with lettuce leads to diarrhea.

**[Diet Therapy Recommended by the Doctor]**

◎ *Usage and dosage of Fengmi (Mel) in diet therapy*

Fengmi (Mel) is sweet and placid. About 25g are recommended for adults to take with warm water every day, and about 10g for children. It can be boiled with white radish to moisten the lung and relieve cough, and boiled with Gouqizi (Lycii Fructus) to protect the liver, the amount of which is 10–20g.

◎ *What season is Fengmi (Mel) most suitable for taking?*

Fengmi (Mel) can be taken all year round. In spring, Fengmi (Mel) can help relieve fatigue. In summer, Fengmi (Mel) is taken with cold water to cool down. The weather is dry in autumn and winter, so Fengmi (Mel) can nourish yin and moisten dryness.

◎ *How to combine Fengmi (Mel) with other medicinal materials and food ingredients?*

If there is fluid retention in the body, Gansui Banxia Decoction can be used together with Fengmi (Mel); for those who are hard and full below the heart, with fluid retention in the upper body, dry eyes and intestines, Banxia (Pinelliae Rhizoma) and Baishao (Paeoniae Radix Alba) can be combined to eliminate fluid in the upper body and lower it. Fengmi (Mel) can not only restrict the stern nature of Gansui (Kansui Radix), Banxia (Pinelliae Rhizoma) and other medicinals, but also harmonize the qi and blood of the human body, help to eliminate the fluid retention in the body, increase efficiency and reduce toxicity.

In daily life, Fengmi (Mel) Gouqizi (Lycii Fructus) water has a good fire-reducing effect, which can often be used to relieve sores on the mouth and tongue, protect eyes and improve eyesight. Fengmi (Mel) brown sugar water can dilute the stain. Pear Fengmi (Mel) water can Stop coughing and help sober up. Ginger Fengmi (Mel) water can relieve pharyngitis and dysmenorrhea.

### Small experiential recipe

*1. To treat functional constipation*

Fengmi (Mel) 50g, royal jelly 5g. Mix well for for oral taking, once in the morning and once in the evening.

*2. To treat postpartum blood deficiency*

Fengmi (Mel) 50g, milk 50ml, Heizhima (Sesami Semen Nigrum) 25g. Mash Heizhima (Sesami Semen Nigrum), and mix with milk and Fengmi (Mel) for oral taking. Take with warm boiled water on an empty stomach in the morning.

*3. To treat bronchial asthma in children*

Fengmi (Mel) 20g, 2 eggs. Fry eggs, add Fengmi (Mel) in while hot, and eat immediately. Once daily for 2–3 months.

# XI Heye (Nelumbinis Folium)

◎ *Where is the best quality Heye (Nelumbinis Folium) produced?*

China is a high-quality Heye (Nelumbinis Folium) producing area, especially in the West Lake, Hangzhou.

◎ *How to distinguish the quality of Heye (Nelumbinis Folium)?*

Heye (Nelumbinis Folium) with large slices, neat appearance, fresh green color, dry and free from moth-eaten, and dry is regarded as good quality.

◎ *How to preserve Heye (Nelumbinis Folium)?*

The decoction pieces of Heye (Nelumbinis Folium) are divided into dried Heye (Nelumbinis Folium) and fresh Heye (Nelumbinis Folium). Dried Heye (Nelumbinis Folium) can be stored in an airtight container, in a dry and ventilated place away from light. Fresh Heye (Nelumbinis Folium) can be cut off roots, rinsed, scalded with boiling water, drained and put into fresh-keeping bags, and frozen for preservation.

◎ *What is the difference between fresh and dry Heye (Nelumbinis Folium)?*

Fresh Heye (Nelumbinis Folium) has the effects of eliminating fat and facilitating feces excretion and urination. Dry Heye (Nelumbinis Folium) is cooler, and has the effects of clearing summer heat and promoting diuresis, raising yang and stopping diarrhea, removing blood stasis, and stopping bleeding. Dry Heye (Nelumbinis Folium) is more used for medicine, while fresh Heye (Nelumbinis Folium) is more used in the diet.

[Efficacy Told by the Doctor]

◎ *Medicinal properties and efficacy—clearing heat and relieving summer heat, ascending clear and stopping diarrhea*

Heye (Nelumbinis Folium) is slightly bitter and cool. It enters the heart, liver, stomach, and spleen meridians. Heye (Nelumbinis Folium) is cool, can eliminate the pathogen of summer heat, and can also treat diarrhea due to summer heat and dampness. In addition, after being charred, Heye (Nelumbinis Folium) astringes, removes blood stasis, and stops bleeding, which is used for various hemorrhagic diseases and postpartum faintness. Heye (Nelumbinis Folium) is born in a pond, leaves out of silt without staining and grows well in places where water and humidity are scattered, which proves that Heye (Nelumbinis Folium) has a better effect of eliminating dampness. Heye (Nelumbinis Folium) is born in summer and the abovewater part can still stay bright green, so its heat removal effect is also excellent. Heye (Nelumbinis Folium) enters the meridians of the spleen and stomach, and the spleen governs ascending and clearing, while stomach governs descending turbidity. Heye (Nelumbinis Folium) can regulate the function of ascending the clear and descending the turbidity of the spleen and stomach.

◎ *Applicable people—summer heat, diarrhea due to damp pathogen, blood stasis and bleeding*

Heye (Nelumbinis Folium) is mainly suitable for people with diarrhea, excessive blood stasis, or bleeding symptoms due to pathogenic summer heat and dampness.

Patients of summer heat strike present a sudden high fever, dizziness, headache, sweating, dry mouth, thirst, and so on.

Those with diarrhea due to damp pathogen present head as heavy as a bundle, diarrhea, sticky stool, heavy limbs, and so on.

Those with blood stasis present dry and scaly skin, ecchymosis and petechia, dull complexion, cyanotic lips, stabbing and fixed pain.

Those with bleeding have bleeding in the digestive tract, respiratory tract or skin, and excessive menstruation in women.

◎ *Applicable syndrome*

Heye (Nelumbinis Folium) can clear away heat, eliminate dampness, relieve summer heat, stop bleeding and dissipate blood stasis. It can be used for people with affection of pathogenic summer heat and diarrhea due to dampness-heat, and can lower blood sugar level and blood lipid, protect immune organs, enhance immune function, resist cancer and virus, etc. It can also be used for headache, dizziness, body edema, hematochezia, metrorrhagia, hematemesis, epistaxis, postpartum hemorrhage, and other diseases.

◎ *What kinds of people are not suitable for Heye (Nelumbinis Folium)?*

As Heye (Nelumbinis Folium) is bitter and cool, those who are weak in qi and blood and who are thin should take with caution. For those who are weak or have severe deficiency cold of the spleen and stomach, do not take Heye (Nelumbinis Folium) tea too much, otherwise it will easily cause physical discomfort, diarrhea, and even dehydration. Women during menstruation are not allowed to take Heye (Nelumbinis Folium). Heye (Nelumbinis Folium) inhibits tung oil and Fuling (Poria), so they cannot be used together.

**[Diet Therapy Recommended by the Doctor]**

◎ *Usage and dosage of Heye (Nelumbinis Folium) in diet therapy*

Heye (Nelumbinis Folium) is cool and slightly bitter and about 15g can be used every day. Heye (Nelumbinis Folium) porridge cooked with japonica rice and rock sugar, clears away heat and promotes diuresis, lowers blood pressure and blood lipid. It is also added in boiled green tea to lose weight by reducing fat.

◎ *What season is Heye (Nelumbinis Folium) most suitable for taking?*

Heye (Nelumbinis Folium) can be taken all year round, but because of its cool nature, it is the most suitable in summer. It can clear summer heat and promote diuresis, prevent heatstroke or excessive moisture.

◎ *How to combine Heye (Nelumbinis Folium) with other medicinal materials and food ingredients?*

People with "three highs" (hypertension, hyperlipidemia and hyperglycemia) can use Heye (Nelumbinis Folium) with Shanzha (Crataegi Fructus). It can be used together with Aiye (Artemisiae Argyi Folium), Cebaiye (Platycladi Cacumen) and Dihuang (Rehmanniae Radix) to treat hematemesis and epistaxis. It can be used together with Puhuang (Typhae Pollen) and Huangqin (Scutellariae

Radix) to treat hemorrhage.

In daily life, Heye (Nelumbinis Folium) porridge can cool off the summer heat, and lower blood pressure and lipid. With green tea, it can reduce fat to lose weight and detoxify. Combined with white sugar, it can treat diarrhea. Mixed well with sesame oil, it can treat impetigo. With wax gourd, it can clear summer heat, promote urination, and relieve irritability.

**Small experiential recipe**

*1. To treat hypertension and hyperlipidemia*
Fresh Heye (Nelumbinis Folium) 2 pieces, Shanzha (Crataegi Fructus) 50g, and Yiyiren (Coicis Semen) 50g, are cooked as porridge for breakfast or dinner.

*2. To treat obesity*
Fresh Heye (Nelumbinis Folium) 1 piece, laver 20g. Boil the Heye (Nelumbinis Folium) in clear water, remove the residue and get the juice, then pour the juice into the laver and cook together, and take it before meals.

*3. To treat skin miliaria*
Fresh Heye (Nelumbinis Folium) 1 piece and a proper amount of mung beans are boiled together for decoction.

## XII　**Heizhima** (Sesami Semen Nigrum)

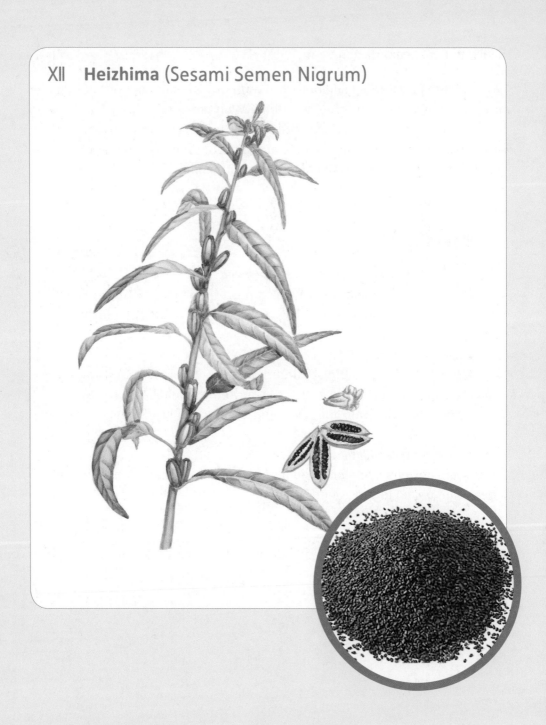

◎ *Where is the best Heizhima (Sesami Semen Nigrum) produced?*

Heizhima (Sesami Semen Nigrum) produced in Zhumadian of Henan Province is regarded as good quality.

◎ *How to distinguish the quality of Heizhima (Sesami Semen Nigrum)?*

Heizhima (Sesami Semen Nigrum) with complete grain, bright black color, no peculiar smell, white color at transverse section which fades after rubbing, and a slightly sweet taste is characteristic of good quality.

◎ *How to preserve Heizhima (Sesami Semen Nigrum)?*

Heizhima (Sesami Semen Nigrum) can be divided into raw and cooked ones. Raw Heizhima (Sesami Semen Nigrum) can be dried and put into a large plastic bucket for sealed preservation. Cooked Heizhima (Sesami Semen Nigrum) should be dried before frying, otherwise it is easy to go mouldy, and can be sealed and refrigerated.

◎ *What is the difference between raw and cooked Heizhima (Sesami Semen Nigrum)?*

Raw Heizhima (Sesami Semen Nigrum) can tonify kidney yin, eliminate stomach fire, and focus on moistening intestines and relaxing bowels. After cooking, it is more easily absorbed by human body so that yin and yang are supplemented together, and the stomach is nourished.

[Efficacy Told by the Doctor]

◎ *Medicinal properties and efficacy—nourishing the liver and kidney, benefiting blood and moistening intestines, promoting defecation*

Heizhima (Sesami Semen Nigrum) is sweet and placid, and belongs to the liver, kidney, and large intestine meridians. It is black and enters the kidney meridian, so it can nouris the liver and kidney. Heizhima (Sesami Semen Nigrum) is an oily crop, containing a lot of fatty substances, and can moisten dryness and treat constipation caused by intestinal dryness and fluid deficiency.

◎ *Applicable people—deficiency of the liver and kidney, blood deficiency, intestinal dryness and constipation*

Heizhima (Sesami Semen Nigrum) is mainly suitable for people with deficiency of liver and kidney yin essence, blood deficiency, intestinal dryness, and constipation, and is mostly used for people with poor constitution, blood deficiency and fluid deficiency, soreness of waist and knees and dry stool.

Patients with deficiency of yin essence in the liver and kidney often present soreness of the waist and knees, dizziness, depression, and dry eyes. Men may have strong yang, causing excess erection, spermatorrhea and premature ejaculation.

People with blood deficiency may have a pale complexion, pale nails, and easy fatigue, while women may have symptoms such as less menstruation and delayed menstruation.

People with constipation usually present difficult defecation, dry stool, which may damage the intestinal collaterals and cause a small amount of bleeding.

◎ *Applicable syndrome*

Heizhima (Sesami Semen Nigrum) can be used for reducing white hair and slight anemia. Heizhima (Sesami Semen Nigrum) contains more than 80% calcium, which can supplement calcium and much potassium, which is beneficial to discharging sodium and lower blood pressure to protect heart health.

◎ *What kinds of people are not suitable for Heizhima (Sesami Semen Nigrum)?*

Because Heizhima (Sesami Semen Nigrum) is rich in vitamin E, people with breast nodules, hyperplasia of mammary glands and breast cysts should eat as little Heizhima (Sesami Semen Nigrum) as possible. Because Heizhima (Sesami

Semen Nigrum) is an oily crop and contain rich fat, which can smooth the intestines and relieve constipation, yet people with frequent diarrhea or with irritable bowel syndrome should eat less Heizhima (Sesami Semen Nigrum). Cooked Heizhima (Sesami Semen Nigrum) is too dry, so it is not suitable for people with internal heat and excessive fire.

[Diet Therapy Recommended by the Doctor]

◎ *Diet therapy usage and dosage of Heizhima (Sesami Semen Nigrum)*

Take 15–20g of Heizhima (Sesami Semen Nigrum) daily. It can be cooked as porridge with japonica rice and Dazao (Jujubae Fructus), or ground into powder to take with Gouqizi (Lycii Fructus).

◎ *What season is Heizhima (Sesami Semen Nigrum) most suitable for taking?*

Heizhima (Sesami Semen Nigrum) can be taken all year round, but it works best in winter. Heizhima (Sesami Semen Nigrum) is black and enters into the kidney, and yang qi is stored in the kidney in winter. At this time, taking Heizhima (Sesami Semen Nigrum) is in line with the four solar terms and the changes of yin, yang, qi and blood of the human body to help reinforce the healthy qi of the human body and strengthen the genuine qi in the kidney. Therefore, taking Heizhima (Sesami Semen Nigrum) in winter is the best way to nourish the kidney.

◎ *How to combine Heizhima (Sesami Semen Nigrum) with other medicinal materials and food ingredients?*

Heizhima (Sesami Semen Nigrum) can be used with Gouqizi (Lycii Fructus) and Shudihuang (Rehmanniae Radix Praeparata) to treat dizziness, blurred vision, insomnia, forgetfulness, soreness and weakness of waist and knees. It cooperates with Heshouwu (Polygoni Multiflori Radix), Sangshen (Mori Fructus) and Gouqizi (Lycii Fructus) to treat white hair. It is fried and ground into powder and then mixed with honey to treat postpartum constipation and habitual constipation.

## Small experiential recipe

### 1. To treat chronic low back pain

30g of Heizhima (Sesami Semen Nigrum) and 30g of the walnut kernel are washed, soaked in 500g white wine, sealed for half a month, and taken twice a day, 15g for each time.

### 2. To treat senile chronic asthma

Heizhima (Sesami Semen Nigrum) 250g, white honey 75g (steamed), ginger juice 5g, rock sugar 75g (mashed and steamed). Dissolve the mashed and steamed rock sugar in Heizhima (Sesami Semen Nigrum) and stir-fry them. After cooling, pour in ginger juice and mix well. Stir-fry again and let them cool. Mix with steamed white honey and put them in a bottle, one teaspoonful in the morning and one teaspoonful in the evening.

### 3. To treat pregnancy constipation

Heizhima (Sesami Semen Nigrum) 60g, almond 5g, and walnut 10g are mashed, steamed with water, and mixed with brown sugar. Take them once every other day and three times a day.

### 4. To treat senile constipation

Heizhima (Sesami Semen Nigrum) 15g, japonica rice 150g and a proper amount of honey. Stir-fry Heizhima (Sesami Semen Nigrum), cook japonica rice with water, and pour Heizhima (Sesami Semen Nigrum) in to cook together. Cool them slightly, add some honey and mix them well. Take them twice a day, once in the morning and once in the evening.

# XIII  **Machixian** (Portulacae Herba)

◎ *Which part of the plant is used as Machixian (Portulacae Herba)?*

The dry aerial part of Portulaceae plant *Portulaca oleracea* L..

◎ *How to distinguish the quality of Machixian (Portulacae Herba)?*

It is better to have a small plant with many leaves, tender texture, and green color.

◎ *How to preserve Machixian (Portulacae Herba)?*

The decoction pieces of Machixian (Portulacae Herba) can be divided into fresh and dried products. Fresh Machixian (Portulacae Herba) can be wrapped in plastic wrap and refrigerated. It can also be scalded with salt boiling water, fished out and drained, dried in the sun, put into a clean plastic bag and stored in a cool place. The dried product should guard againt damp and stored in a cool and dry place, avoiding exposure to sunlight.

◎ *How should Machixian (Portulacae Herba) be used as medicine?*

It is better to use raw Machixian (Portulacae Herba), which can clear heat and detoxify, cool blood, stop bleeding and stop dysentery.

[Efficacy Told by the Doctor]

◎ *Medicinal properties and efficacy—clearing heat and detoxifying, cooling blood and stopping bleeding and dysentery*

Machixian (Portulacae Herba) is slightly acid, cold in nature, slightly odorous, and enters the liver and large intestine meridians. It is cold and slightly acid, which can clear heat and detoxify, cool blood, and stop bleeding. Acid can astringe so it can treat blood dysentery and diarrhea due to heat toxins. Entering the liver meridian, it has the effects of clearing heat and cooling blood, astringing and stopping bleeding, and can treat downward flow of dampness-heat. It can be used externally to treat carbuncle, furuncle, erysipelas, snake bite and eczema.

◎ *Applicable people—downward flow of dampness-heat, blood dysentery due to heat toxin, skin rash*

Machixian (Portulacae Herba) is mainly used for people with excessive heat toxins and dampness-heat, and is mostly used for people suffering from dysentery, tenesmus, hematochezia, metrorrhagia and leakage.

Those with downward flow of dampness-heat mainly present abdominal pain, diarrhea, tenesmus, yellow leucorrhea, short and red urine, damp-heat stranguria and so on.

Those with heat toxins and blood dysentery mainly present high fever, faint, mucopurulent bloody stool, abdominal pain, burning anus, tenesmus, etc.

Those with skin rash mainly have skin eczema, wet sores, yellow pus, and so on.

◎ *Applicable syndrome*

Machixian (Portulacae Herba) has the curative effect of detoxification, and can be used for the dysentery and hematochezia. It can also promote urination and eliminate dampness, used for various types of eczema and wet sore. In addition, it has lipid lowering effect, so it can improve hyperlipidemia.

◎ *What kinds of people are not suitable for Machixian (Portulacae Herba)?*

Machixian (Portulacae Herba) is cold in nature, so people with deficiency cold of the spleen and stomach should not take it. Those with diarrhea due to slippery intestines which belong to deficiency of middle jiao yang qi failing to consolidate should also avoid taking it. Machixian (Portulacae Herba) is cold and smooth, so pregnant women should use it with caution.

**[Diet Therapy Recommended by the Doctor]**

◎ *Usage and dosage of Machixian (Portulacae Herba) in diet therapy*

Machixian (Portulacae Herba) is cold, so generally overeat is not recommemded.

In daily life, 12–16g of dried Machixian (Portulacae Herba) and 35–65g of fresh Machixian (Portulacae Herba) are preferred. About 250–300g of Machixian (Portulacae Herba) can be used to make cold dish, about 300g for congee, and about 80g for scrambled eggs.

◎ *What season is Machixian (Portulacae Herba) most suitable for taking?*

Machixian (Portulacae Herba) is cold in nature and a little acid in flavor, so it is usually taken from March to August.

◎ *How to combine Machixian (Portulacae Herba)medicinal materials and food ingredients?*

Machixian (Portulacae Herba), combined with Huangqin (Scutellariae Radix) and Huanglian (Coptidis Rhizoma), can treat acute tenesmus. It can be used together with Diyu (Sanguisorbae Radix), Huaijiao (Sophorae Fructus) and Fengweicao (Petridis Multifidae Herba Herba) to treat hemorrhoidal bleeding due to downward flow of dampness-heat. With Qiancao (Rubiae Radix et Rhizoma), Zhumagen (Boehmeriae Radix) and Cebaiye (Platycladi Cacumen), it can treat blood heat bleeding, metrorrhagia and metrostaxis, or it can be taken alone when mashed.

In daily life, Machixian (Portulacae Herba) can be combined with Qianshi (Euryales Semen) and lean meat to clear heat and detoxify, eliminate dampness and stop leukorrhagia. Go with white sugar and vinegar, it can play the role of deworming. It is fried with eggs to clear heat and detoxify to stop dysentery, replenish qi and tonify deficiency, and is used for damp-heat chronic dysentery. It is cooked as porridge with japonica rice to treat dysentery, hematochezia and damp-heat diarrhea. It can also be mashed with fresh lotus root for juice to clear heat and stop bleeding.

**Small experiential recipe**

*1. To treat damp-heat or heat toxins dysentery and diarrhea*
Machixian (Portulacae Herba) 30g (double the amount for the fresh herb), rice 100g, and a proper amount of white sugar are cooked as porridge, and boiled twice, one dose a day, and take it for 5 consecutive days.

**2. To treat hematochezia caused by the lesions of the large intestines**

Fresh Machixian (Portulacae Herba) 100g, Huaihua (Sophorae Flos) 30g, japonica rice 100g and brown sugar 20g are cooked as porridge. Huaihua (Sophorae Flos) should be added later. Take it twice, once in the morning and once in the evening.

**3. To treat leukorrhea with reddish discharge**

Machixian (Portulacae Herba) 250g, 2 eggs. Mashed Machixian (Portulacae Herba), and mix with egg white, and taken with boiling water. Take it twice daily.

**4. To treat hookworm disease in children**

Machixian (Portulacae Herba) 200–250g, vinegar 30g, and proper amount of white sugar. Decoct Machixian (Portulacae Herba) to get the concentrated juice without dregs, then add vinegar and white sugar, and mix well. Drink it once or twice on an empty stomach for 3 consecutive days. If it is required to take again, take it after half a month.

# XIV  **Pugongying** (Taraxaci Herba)

## [Drug Selection by the Pharmacist]

◎ *Which part of the plant is used as Pugongying (Taraxaci Herba)?*

The dry herb if Compositae plant *Taraxacum mongolicum* Hand-Mazz, *Taraxacum borealisinense* Kitam. or several other *Taraxacum* plants.

◎ *Where is high quality Pugongying (Taraxaci Herba) produced?*

The quality of Pugongying (Taraxaci Herba) produced in Hebei and Sichuan and is the best.

◎ *How to distinguish the quality of Pugongying (Taraxaci Herba)?*

It is better to have Pugongying (Taraxaci Herba) with many leaves, gray-green color and roots.

◎ *How to preserve Pugongying (Taraxaci Herba)?*

Wash the fresh Pugongying (Taraxaci Herba) and dry it in a ventilated place naturally, or drain and refrigerate it. Defrost it when serving. Dry Pugongying (Taraxaci Herba) can be placed directly in a cool and ventilated place, protected from light.

◎ *In terms of efficacy, what is the difference among roots and leaves of Pugongying (Taraxaci Herba)?*

Pugongying (Taraxaci Herba) can be used as medicine, with its roots focusing on detoxifying and clearing heat of the liver, leaves on anti-inflammation and detoxification, which are indicated for gingival irritation or oral ulcer.

## [Efficacy Told by the Doctor]

◎ *Medicinal properties and efficacy—clearing heat and detoxifying, reducing swelling and dissipating masses, promoting urination and relieving stranguria*

Pugongying (Taraxaci Herba) is cold, bitter, and sweet, and enters liver and stomach meridians. Its cold nature can clear heat and detoxify, and can be used for carbuncles, furuncles, breast carbuncle, lung carbuncle, intestinal carbuncle, and scrofula. It can clear liver, improve eyesight, reduce swelling and resolve masses, and treat red eyes, swelling, and pain caused by upward flaming of liver fire. Its bitter taste can reduce dryness, and treat damp-heat jaundice, heat stranguria and astringent pain. In addition, the juice can be used as eye drop. It can also be applied externally to treat carbuncle and furuncle.

◎ *Applicable people—internal and external heat, toxin, sore and carbuncle, damp-heat jaundice and stranguria*

Pugongying (Taraxaci Herba) is mainly cold and bitter, which is mainly used for the syndromes of excessive internal and external heat toxins and dampness-heat in the lower jiao. It is mostly used for people with body heat and irritability.

People with internal and external heat toxins often present carbuncles, furuncles, breast carbuncle, lung carbuncle with vomiting pus, sore throat, venomous snake bite, etc.

People with damp-heat jaundice, is often manifested by fever, yellow eyes, yellow body and yellow urine.

People with stranguria is often manifested by short, red and painful urination, and endless dripping.

◎ *Applicable syndrome*

Pugongying (Taraxaci Herba) has the effect of clearing away heat and detoxification. It can be used to treat sore throat caused by colds, and can also be used for chronic gastritis, enteritis, jaundice and so on.

◎ *What kinds of people are not suitable for Pugongying (Taraxaci Herba)?*

Pugongying (Taraxaci Herba) is cold, and people with spleen and stomach deficiency and yang deficiency constitution, women with uterus cold and people with yin cold syndrome are not suitable for eating it. In addition, excessive dosage will lead to symptoms such as epigastric pain, and even diarrhea in severe cases, so attention should be paid to the clinical application.

◎ *Usage and dosage of Pugongying (Taraxaci Herba) in diet therapy*

The daily dosage of fresh Pugongying (Taraxaci Herba) for adults should not exceed 60g, and that for children should be halved; dried Pugongying (Taraxaci Herba) should not exceed 12g per day for adults and a half for children. Pugongying (Taraxaci Herba) is rich in edible methods, including stir-frying, cold dish, porridge or stuffing.

◎ *What season is Pugongying (Taraxaci Herba) most suitable for taking?*

Pugongying (Taraxaci Herba) is cold, and it is best to take it when it is hot in summer and autumn. Pugongying (Taraxaci Herba) can also be taken in spring, which helps improve immunity.

◎ *How to combine Pugongying (Taraxaci Herba) with other medicinal materials and food ingredients?*

Pugongying (Taraxaci Herba) can be used with Gualou (Trichosanthis Fructus) and Jinyinhua (Lonicerae Japonicae Flos) to treat swelling and pain of breast carbuncle. It can be used with Jinyinhua (Lonicerae Japonicae Flos), Yejuhua (Chrysanthemi Indici Flos) and Zihuadiding (Violae Herba) to treat carbuncle, swelling and furuncle. Combined with Dahuang (Rhei Radix et Rhizoma), Mudanpi (Moutan Cortex), and Taoren (Persicae Semen), it can treat intestinal carbuncle and abdominal pain. It can be used with Yuxingcao (Houttuyniae Herba), Dongguaren (Benincasae Semen) and Lugen (Phragmitis Rhizoma) to treat lung carbuncle and pus vomiting. It is combined with Xiakucao (Prunellae Spica), Lianqiao (Forsythiae Fructus) and Zhebeimu (Fritillariae Thunbergii Bulbus) to treat scrofula. It can also be combined with Banlangen (Isatidis Radix) and Xuanshen (Scrophulariae Radix) to treat sore throat.

In daily diet therapy, cooked with pork or beef, etc., it has the effects of clearing heat and detoxifying, nourishing yin, and protecting yang. Go with corn core to be taken as tea, and it can treat hot stranguria and short red urine. Fried with eggs, it can relieve irritability, threatened miscarriage and sore throat caused by wind-heat.

*1. To treat excessive heat toxins and internal and external swelling*

Fresh Pugongying (Taraxaci Herba) 35g and japonica rice 150g are cooked as porridge to take at meal time.

*2. To treat cough with yellow and thick phlegm*

Fresh Pugongying (Taraxaci Herba) 60g and pork 200g are cooked for eaing. Once a day.

*3. To treat beriberi*

Fresh Pugongying (Taraxaci Herba) 15–35g, boil first and then have feet massage in the warm water, twice a day, once for 15–30 minutes. Fresh Pugongying (Taraxaci Herba) can be mashed for external use to sterilize and treat beriberi.

# XV  **Lianzi** (Nelumbinis Semen)

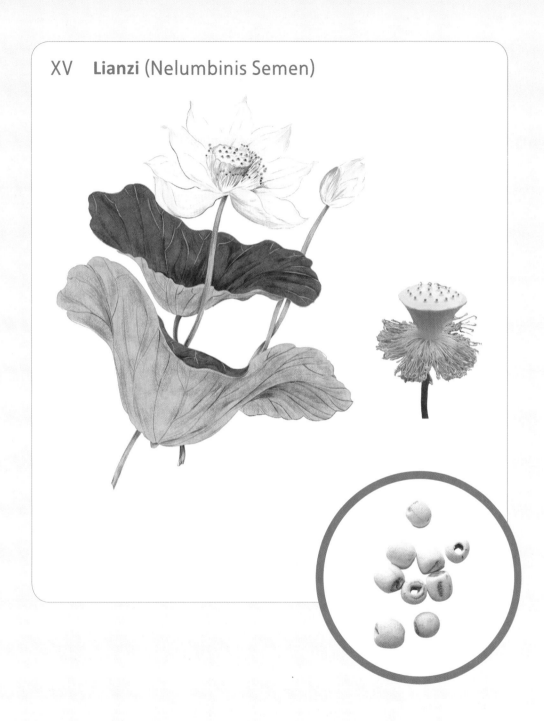

◎ *Which part of Lianzi (Nelumbinis Semen) is used for medicine?*

The dry and mature seed of the Nymphaeaceae plant *Nelumbo nucifera* Gaertn. is used as Lianzi (Nelumbinis Semen), with its germ removed.

◎ *Where is high quality Lianzi (Nelumbinis Semen) is produced?*

Jianlian produced in Jianning County, Fujian Province, Xuanlian produced in Xuanping, Wuyi County, Zhejiang Province, Bailian produced in Guangchang County, Jiangxi Province, and Xianglian produced in Xiangtan City, Hunan Province are of good quality.

◎ *How to distinguish the quality of Lianzi (Nelumbinis Semen)?*

It is better to be large, full, neat, and free of impurities and peculiar smell, and light yellow and shiny in color.

◎ *How to preserve Lianzi (Nelumbinis Semen)?*

Mature Lianzi (Nelumbinis Semen) is picked with the green hull reserved, and stored in the refrigerator. It can also be dried and stored in an airtight container or a plastic bag.

[Efficacy Told by the Doctor]

◎ *Medicinal properties and efficacy—tonifying the spleen to stop diarrhea, stopping leukorrhagia, tonifying the kidney to astringe essence, nourishing the heart and calming minds*

Lianzi (Nelumbinis Semen) is sweet, astringent, and not biased. It enters the spleen, kidney, and heart meridians. It is sweet and neutral, enters the heart and kidney meridians, can nourish the heart, benefit the kidney, calm the minds, restore interaction between the heart and the kidney, and treat palpitation and insomnia. It enters the spleen meridian, can tonify the spleen and stop diarrhea, and treat diarrhea due to spleen deficiency. It can astringe discharge and stop leukorrhagia, and treat female leukorrhagia. Therefore, the taste is sweet and astringent, so it can astringe and stop seminal emission.

◎ *Applicable people—diarrhea due to spleen deficiency, deficiency of the spleen and kidney, and disharmony between the heart and kidney*

Lianzi (Nelumbinis Semen) is mainly suitable for people with spleen and kidney deficiency and heart and kidney disharmony and is mostly used for diarrhea, vexation, palpitation, insomnia, female leukorrhagia and male spermatorrhea due to spleen deficiency. In addition, Lianzi (Nelumbinis Semen) belongs to both medicine and food, and people without diseases take proper Lianzi (Nelumbinis Semen) daily on ordinary days will have good healthcare effect.

Those with diarrhea due to spleen deficiency mainly present fatigue of limbs, diarrhea, and a sallow complexion.

Those with deficiency of the spleen and kidney mainly present soreness and weakness of the waist and knees, clear leukorrhea in women, spermatorrhea and night emission in men, etc.

Those with disharmony between the heart and kidney mainly present asthenia vexation, palpitation, insomnia, dizziness, forgetfulness, tinnitus, and so on.

◎ *Applicable syndrome*

Lianzi (Nelumbinis Semen) has the effect of tonifying the spleen and kidney. It can be used to treat diarrhea and fatigue caused by spleen and kidney deficiency. It can also nourish the heart and calm the nerves to treat palpitations and insomnia.

◎ *What kinds of people are not suitable for Lianzi (Nelumbinis Semen)?*

Because Lianzi (Nelumbinis Semen) is sweet and astringent and has strong astringent effects, people with dry stool caused by intestinal dryness and fluid deficiency should not eat it.

◎ *Usage and dosage of Lianzi (Nelumbinis Semen) in diet therapy*

Lianzi (Nelumbinis Semen) is sweet and astringent in taste and not biased. Generally 15–30g is used for daily serving. It can be used for preparing congee, soup and other dishes.

◎ *What season is Lianzi (Nelumbinis Semen) most suitable for taking?*

Lianzi (Nelumbinis Semen) has mild medicinal properties, so it can be taken all year round without confinement to the changes of four seasons.

◎ *How to combine Lianzi (Nelumbinis Semen) with other medicinal materials and food ingredients?*

Lianzi (Nelumbinis Semen) is combined with Renshen (Ginseng Radix et Rhizoma), Fuling (Poria), and Baizhu (Atractylodis Macrocephalae Rhizoma) to treat prolonged diarrhea and anorexia due to spleen deficiency. Combined with Shanyao (Dioscoreae Rhizoma), Baizhu (Atractylodis Macrocephalae Rhizoma), and Fuling (Poria), it can treat leucorrhea due to spleen deficiency. Combined with Shanyao (Dioscoreae Rhizoma), Qianshi (Euryales Semen) and Shanzhuyu (Corni Fructus), it can treat spleen and kidney deficiency, clear leucorrhea, soreness and weakness of waist and knees. To treat spermatorrhea and night emission, it can be used with Longgu (Draconis Os) and Qianshi (Euryales Semen). To treat palpitation and insomnia, it can be combined with Suanzaoren (Ziziphi Spinosae Semen), Fuling (Poria), and Yuanzhi (Polygalae Radix).

In daily life, soup can be made together with tremella and rock sugar to nourish yin and moisten the lung, nourish the stomach and promote fluid production. With Baihe (Lilii Bulbus) and Gouqizi (Lycii Fructus), it clears the heart and remove heat. Cooked with Baihe (Lilii Bulbus) and lean pork as congee, it tonifies the spleen and lung, and boosts qi.

*1. To treat palpitation, vexation, and insomnia*

Lianzi (Nelumbinis Semen) 15g, brown sugar 10g, glutinous rice 150g. Remove lotus plumule, cook as porridge, once a day and take it at the meal time.

*2. To treat cough due to spleen and lung qi deficiency in the middle-aged and elderly people*

Lianzi (Nelumbinis Semen) 25g, Baihe (Lilii Bulbus) 25g, lean pork 300g. Well cook with proper amount of various seasonings as broth, and take it twice a week.

*3. To treat female leukorrhagia*

Lianzi (Nelumbinis Semen) 15g, Baiguo (Ginkgo Semen) 20g and 1 black-bone chicken (about 600g). Put Lianzi (Nelumbinis Semen) and Baiguo (Ginkgo Semen) into the belly of the chicken, add some seasonings, and stew them in clear water. Once a day.

*4. To treat anemia*

Lianzi (Nelumbinis Semen) 25g, Longyanrou (Longan Arillus) 15g, glutinous rice 50g. Boil for porridge, and take it warm, twice a day.

*5. To treat dizziness due to blood deficiency*

Lianzi (Nelumbinis Semen) 30g, Daozao (Jujubae Fructus) 15 pieces, Longyanrou (Longan Arillus) 20g, peanuts 20g. Boil them in water and eat twice a day.

# XVI  **Jiang** (Shengjiang, Zingiberis Rhizoma Recens; Ganjiang, Zingiberis Rhizoma)

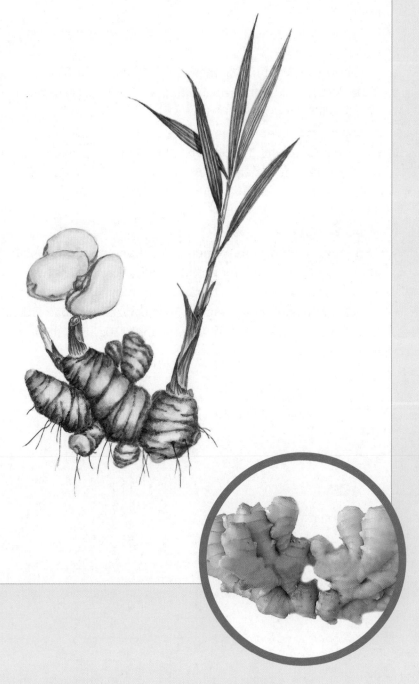

## [Drug Selection by the Pharmacist]

◎ *Can ginger skin be used as medicine?*

The rhizome of Zingiberaceae family plant *Zingiber officinale* Rosc. is used as medicine, and is used with skin. The skin of ginger can also be used as medicine alone.

◎ *Where is the best ginger produced?*

It is produced in most parts of China, and ginger produced in Sichuan and Shandong is the most famous. Ganjiang (Zingiberis Rhizoma) grown in Sichuan is of the best quality.

◎ *How to distinguish the quality of ginger?*

Shengjiang (Zingiberis Rhizoma Recens) is better if it is large, plump, and tender. Ganjiang (Zingiberis Rhizoma) white in color, ample in powder, and spicy in taste is regarded as good quality.

◎ *How to preserve ginger?*

Shengjiang (Zingiberis Rhizoma Recens) should be placed in a cool and humid place, or buried in wet sand to prevent frostbite. Ganjiang (Zingiberis Rhizoma) can be stored in a cool place.

◎ *What's the difference between Shengjiang (Zingiberis Rhizoma Recens) and Ganjiang (Zingiberis Rhizoma)?*

Shengjiang (Zingiberis Rhizoma Recens) has a good effect of relieving exterior syndrome and dispelling cold, while Ganjiang (Zingiberis Rhizoma) has a good effect of warming the middle and dispelling cold. And ginger peel has a strong effect on diuresis and detumescence.

## [Efficacy Told by the Doctor]

◎ *Medicinal properties and efficacy—warming the lung and dispelling cold*

Shengjiang (Zingiberis Rhizoma Recens) is pungent and warm. It enters

Section 1   Chinese Medicinals Used for Both Medicine and Food   237 the lung, spleen and stomach meridians, so it can relieve exterior syndrome, dispel cold, warm the lung, relieve cough, warm the middle and stop vomiting. However, Ganjiang (Zingiberis Rhizoma) is hotter and has good functions of warming the middle, dispelling cold, returning yang and dredging veins. In addition, Ganjiang (Zingiberis Rhizoma) also has a certain detoxification effect, which can relieve food poisonings such as fish and crab, and can be used to process Banxia (Pinelliae Rhizoma) and Tiannanxing (Arisaematis Rhizoma) to reduce their toxicity.

◎ *Applicable people—yang deficiency constitution, spleen and stomach deficiency cold*

Ginger can be eaten by the general population. It is especially suitable for people with yang deficiency of spleen and stomach and weak constitution and is mostly used for those who are always afraid of cold and easy to catch a cold, and those with deficiency cold of stomach and intestines.

For exogenous wind-cold patients, they mainly present aversion to cold, stuffy nose, clear nasal discharge, headache, body pain, or cough.

For people with deficiency cold of the spleen and stomach, they mainly present dull pain in stomach, vomiting, abdominal pain and diarrhea, and poor appetite.

◎ *Applicable syndrome*

Ginger can be used for arthritis, toothache, severe vomiting, acute gastroenteritis, gastric and duodenal ulcer, acute intestinal obstruction, ascariasis, infantile diarrhea, acute bacillary dysentery, malaria, bedsore and other diseases belonging to the above mentioned syndomes, as well as poisoning first aid and motion sickness treatment.

◎ *What kinds of people are not suitable for ginger?*

Because ginger is warm, it is not suitable for people with yin deficiency, internal heat and excessive pathogenic heat. At the same time, because it tastes pungent and spicy, pregnant women should use it with caution.

◎ *Usage and dosage of ginger in diet therapy*

Ginger for diet therapy can be drunk with tea, with peeled Shengjiang (Zingiberis Rhizoma Recens) 5–10g. For home meals such as stir-frying, cooking soup, porridge, etc., 30–60g of fresh ginger can be used, and 3–10g of Ganjiang (Zingiberis Rhizoma) can be used with other condiments. Ginger should not be taken too much at a time.

◎ *What season is ginger most suitable for taking?*

Ginger can be eaten every day, but it should not be used much in autumn. Autumn is dry, and dryness hurts the lung. Shengjiang (Zingiberis Rhizoma Recens) is pungent, warm and dispersing, so it will purge lung qi.

◎ *How to combine ginger with other medicinal materials and food ingredients?*

Ginger is pungent, dispersing and has a warm-dredging function, but its effect is weak. It is used with pungent and warm exterior-relieving medicinals such as Guizhi (Cinnamomi Ramulus) and Qianghuo (Notopterygii Rhizoma et Radix) when it is used for common cold with the wind-cold syndrome. For those with excessive phlegm, cough, aversion to cold, headache, it usually go with Mahuang (Ephedrae Herba) and Kuxingren (Armeniacae Semen Amarum). It should be used together with interior-warming and qi-tonifying medicinals such as Gaoliangjiang (Alpiniae Officinarum Rhizoma), Hujiao (Piperis Fructus), Dangshen (Codonopsis Radix) and Baizhu (Atractylodis Macrocephalae Rhizoma) to treat cold syndrome of spleen and stomach. It is most suitable for vomiting due to a cold stomach and can be combined with stomach-warming and antiemetic medicinals such as Gaoliangjiang (Alpiniae Officinarum Rhizoma) and Doukou (Amomi Fructus Rotundus).

In cuisine, it can be matched with cool foods, such as bitter gourd, water chestnut, Baihe (Lilii Bulbus), grapefruit, pear, etc. Ginger is warm, which can prevent the cold in the body from aggravating. It can also be used with hot foods such as mutton. Mutton enriches blood and warms yang; Shengjiang (Zingiberis Rhizoma Recens) relieves pain, dispels wind and dampness, dispels fishy smell, and enhances the function of warming yang and dispelling cold.

◎ *How to choose Shengjiang (Zingiberis Rhizoma Recens) and Ganjiang (Zingiberis Rhizoma) as a diet therapy?*

Shengjiang (Zingiberis Rhizoma Recens) and Ganjiang (Zingiberis Rhizoma) are both tubers of ginger, which have the diet therapy effect of dispelling cold and warming the lung. Shengjiang (Zingiberis Rhizoma Recens) has great divergent power and sweating effect, so it is more suitable for exogenous factors and has a good effect of invigorating the spleen and stimulating appetite. Ganjiang (Zingiberis Rhizoma) is more pungent and warmer, which can warm the middle and dispel cold, and restore yang to dredge the pulse. It is better to treat cold pain, vomiting, diarrhea, cold limbs, and dysmenorrhea in women.

**Small experiential recipe**

*1. To treat cold and cough*

10g of tea and 10g of peeled and sliced Shengjiang (Zingiberis Rhizoma Recens) are decocted in water and taken after meals.

*2. To treat cold dysmenorrhea*

Ganjiang (Zingiberis Rhizoma) 30g, Dazao (Jujubae Fructus) 30g, brown sugar 30g. Wash and slice Ganjiang (Zingiberis Rhizoma), wash and remove the core of Dazao (Jujubae Fructus), and decoct with brown sugar.

Or shred 20g of Shengjiang (Zingiberis Rhizoma Recens), proper amount of brown sugar, boil them with a cover for 3 minutes, and take it warm as tea.

*3. To treat vomiting due to stomach cold*

Juice Shengjiang (Zingiberis Rhizoma Recens), add hot water and honey, mix well and drink.

# XVII Dazao (Jujubae Fructus)

◎ *Which part of the plant is used as Dazao (Jujubae Fructus)?*

The mature fruit of Rhamnaceae plant *Ziziphus jujuba* Mill. is used as medicine.

◎ *Where is the best Dazao (Jujubae Fructus) produced?*

Dazao (Jujubae Fructus) produced in Shandong and Henan has the best quality.

◎ *How to distinguish the quality of Dazao (Jujubae Fructus)?*

Dazao (Jujubae Fructus) is better with large, uniform and fleshy fruit, lustrous color and sweet taste.

◎ *How to preserve Dazao (Jujubae Fructus)?*

Fresh Dazao (Jujubae Fructus) is suitable for preservation after drying, and can be placed in a dry and cool place.

[Efficacy Told by the Doctor]

◎ *Medicinal properties and efficacy—tonifying and calming the mind*

Dazao (Jujubae Fructus) is sweet and warm and has a tonic effect, especially good at nourishing blood to calm the mind.

◎ *Applicable people—peaceful constitution and yin deficiency constitution*

Dazao (Jujubae Fructus) is suitable for ordinary people to keep healthy at ordinary times, especially for those with spleen deficiency, blood deficiency, hysteria of women, insomnia and night sweat due to yin deficiency.

Patients with spleen deficiency mainly present poor diet, emaciation, burnout and fatigue, loose stool and so on.

Patients with blood deficiency are mainly manifested by pale complexion, pale lip, pale nail, withered hair, dizziness, numbness in limbs, palpitation, and so on.

Patients with hysteria and insomnia are mainly manifested by trance, crying and laughing hysterically, emotional fluctuations, vexation, insomnia, forgetfulness, and so on.

◎ *Applicable syndrome*

Dazao (Jujubae Fructus) can be used daily to improve immunity, protect the liver and prevent cardiovascular diseases and anemia. For cardiovascular diseases, anemia, insomnia, emotional depression and other diseases that have occurred, it also has a good curative effect.

◎ *What kinds of people are not suitable for Dazao (Jujubae Fructus)?*

Because Dazao (Jujubae Fructus) is tonic, people with damp-heat and phlegm-dampness constitution are not suitable for taking.

**[Diet Therapy Recommended by the Doctor]**

◎ *Usage and dosage of jujube in diet therapy*

Dazao (Jujubae Fructus) is sweet and gentle in medicinal properties. It is used for daily porridge and soup cooking, and the dosage can be adjusted according to needs, ranging from 30 to 100g, replacing tea with 10 to 15g.

◎ *What season is jujube most suitable for taking?*

Dazao (Jujubae Fructus) can be taken all year round, because it has nourishing effect, so it is especially suitable for health preservation in winter.

◎ *How to combine Dazao (Jujubae Fructus) with other medicinal materials and food ingredients?*

Dazao (Jujubae Fructus) has mild medicinal properties and can be matched with various medicinal materials. Baizhu (Atractylodis Macrocephalae Rhizoma) and Renshen (Ginseng Radix et Rhizoma) are often added for invigorating the middle and benefiting qi, especially when qi deficiency is obvious. To treat hysteria, etc., it is often combined with wheat and Gancao (Glycyrrhizae Radix et Rhizoma). For the treatment of insomnia it is often compatible with Huangqi (Astragali Radix), Danggui (Angelicae Sinensis Radix), Yuanzhi (Polygalae Radix), Shengdihuang (Rehmanniae Radix) and Longyanrou (Longan Arillus). In addition, Dazao (Jujubae Fructus) is used with some medicinals with strong or toxic properties, and has the effect of protecting stomach qi and relieving their toxic properties.

In daily cuisine, it is often matched with Baihe (Lilii Bulbus), Fuling (Poria), Danggui (Angelicae Sinensis Radix) and Longyanrou (Longan Arillus) to strengthen the effects of tonifying, nourishing blood and calming the mind.

## Small experiential recipe

### 1. Daily health preservation and blood enrichment

Wash 100g of Dazao (Jujubae Fructus) and boil them in a pot, then simmer them for 15–20 minutes, and drink the juice.

### 2. To treat anemia

Dazao (Jujubae Fructus) 50g, ginger 5g, brown sugar 10g. Dazao (Jujubae Fructus) and ginger are put into a casserole. Add some water, simmer for half a minute, add some brown sugar and mix them well.

# Section 2
## Chinese Medicinals Used for Healthcare Food

I **Huangqi** (Astragali Radix)

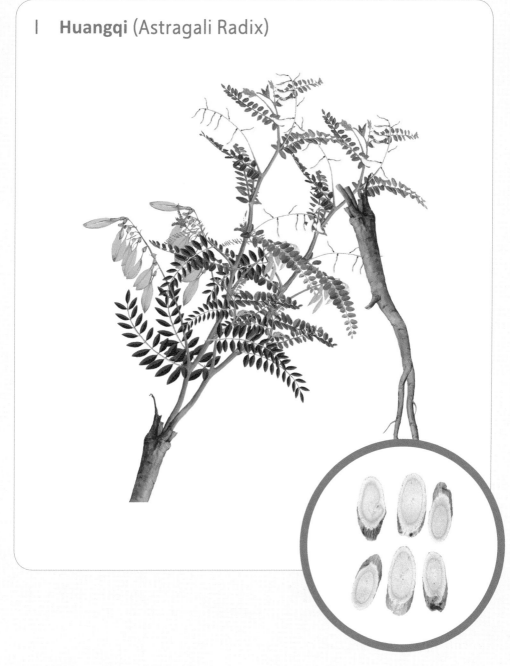

◎ *Which part of the plant is used as Huangqi (Astragali Radix)?*

The root of Leguminosae plant *Astragalus membranaceus* (Fisch.) Bge. var. *mongholicus* (Bge.) Hsiao or *Astragalus membranaceus* (Fisch.) Bge. is used as medicine.

◎ *Where is the best Huangqi (Astragali Radix) produced?*

The quality of Huangqi (Astragali Radix) produced in Inner Mongolia, Shanxi and Heilongjiang is the best.

◎ *How to distinguish the quality of Huangqi (Astragali Radix)?*

It is better to have strong roots, few wrinkles, firm and soft quality, sufficient powder and sweet taste.

◎ *How to preserve Huangqi (Astragali Radix)?*

It can be placed in a dry and cool place.

◎ *What is the difference between raw Huangqi (Astragali Radix) and honey-fried Huangqi (Astragali Radix)?*

The decoction pieces of Huangqi (Astragali Radix) are divided into raw Huangqi (Astragali Radix) and honey-fried Huangqi (Astragali Radix). The former has a good effect of invigorating qi and consolidating the exterior, while the latter has a good effect of invigorating the spleen and stomach.

[Efficacy Told by the Doctor]

◎ *Medicinal properties and efficacy—invigorating the spleen and tonifying the middle, raising yang and lifting the sunken, invigorating qi to consolidate the exterior, promoting urination, dispelling toxin and promoting granulation*

Huangqi (Astragali Radix) is warm and sweet in nature, belongs to the spleen and lung, and has a good effect of strengthening the spleen and benefiting the lung. In addition, it also has a certain effect of invigorating qi and blood, and can be used in combination with blood activating medicinals to treat arthralgia and stroke sequelae.

◎ *Applicable people—weak spleen qi, spontaneous sweating due to lung deficiency, difficult ulceration of sores and ulcers*

Huangqi (Astragali Radix) is mainly suitable for people with spleen and lung and qi deficiency, and is mostly used for people with a thin body, shortness of breath, unwillingness to talk, cough, asthma, spontaneous sweating, fatigue, edema, and less urine.

People with weak spleen qi as the main syndrome are mainly manifested by tiredness and fatigue, reduced appetite, loose stool, indigestion, abdominal pain and diarrhea.

Those with weak lung qi mainly present chronic cough and asthma, shortness of breath, trance, fatigue, spontaneous sweating, and excessive urination.

Those with deficiency of qi and blood as the main syndrome mainly present pale complexion, unwillingness to talk, reduced appetite, spontaneous sweating, fatigue, and refractory ulcers.

◎ *Applicable syndrome*

Huangqi (Astragali Radix) can be used to treat allergic rhinitis, chronic rhinitis, upper respiratory tract infection, angina pectoris, osteoporosis, arthritis, chronic nephritis, chronic hepatitis, asthma in children, coronary heart disease, and postpartum non-infectious fever which belong to syndromes of spleen qi deficiency, lung qi deficiency, qi and blood deficiency.

◎ *What kinds of people are not suitable for Huangqi (Astragali Radix)?*

Because Huangqi (Astragali Radix) is slightly sweet and warm, and has the function of invigorating qi and raising yang, it is not suitable for people with cough due to exogenous wind-heat pathogen, who are afraid of heat and like cold, have a heat stomach and constipation, and like to drink cold water.

If there is intolerance of heat, dry throat and constipation after taking

Huangqi (Astragali Radix), stop using it, and take Huanglian (Coptidis Rhizoma) water appropriately to relieve symptoms.

◎ *Usage and dosage of Huangqi (Astragali Radix) in diet therapy*

Huangqi (Astragali Radix) is sweet and slightly warm, and 5–15g can be used as a substitute for tea in daily life. 10–30g of decoction pieces can be used for home meals such as stir-frying, cooking soup, porridge, etc.

◎ *What season is Huangqi (Astragali Radix) most suitable for taking?*

Huangqi (Astragali Radix) can be taken all year round, because it has the function of invigorating qi and raising yang, especially in autumn and winter.

◎ *How to combine Huangqi (Astragali Radix) with other medicinal materials and food ingredients?*

Huangqi (Astragali Radix) is sweet and slightly warm, and it often assists Renshen (Ginseng Radix et Rhizoma) or Baizhu (Atractylodis Macrocephalae Rhizoma) to enhance its effect of invigorating the spleen and tonifying middle jiao. It is often combined with Ziwan (Asteris Radix et Rhizoma), Kuandonghua (Farfarae Flos) and Kuxingren (Armeniacae Semen Amarum) to treat deficiency of lung qi, chronic cough and asthma, shortness of breath, exhaustion and spontaneous sweating.

In daily cooking, it is often combined with ingredients such as Danggui (Angelicae Sinensis Radix), Baizhu (Atractylodis Macrocephalae Rhizoma), and Fuling (Poria) to strengthen the spleen and invigorate qi. For cooking porridge it is often made with Yiyiren (Coicis Semen), Shanyao (Dioscoreae Rhizoma), etc., to strengthen the spleen and invigorate qi. For making soup it is often combined with Dangshen (Codonopsis Radix), Kuxingren (Armeniacae Semen Amarum), Fangfeng (Saposhnikoviae Radix), etc.

◎ *How to choose Huangqi (Astragali Radix) and Renshen (Ginseng Radix et Rhizoma) as a diet therapy?*

Huangqi (Astragali Radix) and Renshen (Ginseng Radix et Rhizoma) are both sweet and warm, which have the diet therapy effects of invigorating qi, promoting fluid and blood production. They are often used together to improve the curative effect of each other. Compared with Renshen (Ginseng Radix et Rhizoma), Huangqi (Astragali Radix) can promote diuresis and reduce swelling. Therefore, it is more appropriate to choose Huangqi (Astragali Radix) if there is deficiency of spleen and lung, edema and less urine.

## Small experiential recipe

### 1. To treat chronic rhinitis

Huangqi (Astragali Radix) 15g, Baizhu (Atractylodis Macrocephalae Rhizoma) 12g, Fangfeng (Saposhnikoviae Radix) 10g. The above ingregients are decocted, and taken warm. Once in the morning and once in the evening.

### 2. To treat osteoporosis

Huangqi (Astragali Radix) 30g, Guizhi (Cinnamomi Ramulus) 10g, Baishao (Paeoniae Radix Alba) 15g, Shengjiang (Zingiberis Rhizoma Recens) 3 slices, Dazao (Jujubae Fructus) 12 pieces. The above ingredients are cooked for soup, and taken warm. Once in the morning and once in the evening.

# ‖ **Danggui** (Angelicae Sinensis Radix)

[Drug Selection by the Pharmacist]

◎ *Which part of the plant is used as Danggui (Angelicae Sinensis Radix)?*

The root of Umbelliferae plant *Angelica sinensis* (Oliv.) Diels is used as medicine.

◎ *Where is the best Danggui (Angelicae Sinensis Radix) produced?*

Minxian County in the southeast of Gansu Province has more output and better quality. It is also grown in Shaanxi, Sichuan, Yunnan, Hubei Provinces.

◎ *How to distinguish the quality of Danggui (Angelicae Sinensis Radix)?*

Thick, long, oily and plump main root, with yellow and white color at transverse section, and strong fragrance is regarded as good quality.

◎ *How to preserve Danggui (Angelicae Sinensis Radix)?*

Danggui (Angelicae Sinensis Radix) slices can be placed in a dry and cool place.

◎ *What is the difference between raw Danggui (Angelicae Sinensis Radix) and wine-fried Danggui (Angelicae Sinensis Radix)?*

The decoction pieces of Danggui (Angelicae Sinensis Radix) are divided into raw Danggui (Angelicae Sinensis Radix) and wine-fried Danggui (Angelicae Sinensis Radix). The former has a good effect on enriching blood and nourishing blood, while the latter has a good effect on promoting blood circulation and enriching blood.

[Efficacy Told the by Doctor]

◎ *Medicinal properties and efficacy—enriching blood and regulating menstruation, promoting blood circulation and relieving pain, moistening intestines and relieving constipation*

Danggui (Angelicae Sinensis Radix) is sweet, pungent and warm, and has a tonic effect on the liver, heart and spleen. It can replenish blood and regulate menstruation, and treat scanty menstruation caused by blood deficiency. Its medicinal properties are pungent and warm, which can promote blood circulation and relieve pain, and treat the pain caused by blood stasis. In addition, it also has a certain moisturizing and laxative effect, which can treat intestinal dryness and constipation.

◎ *Applicable people—yin deficiency constitution, dry throat, chronic cough, vexation, insomnia*

Danggui (Angelicae Sinensis Radix) is mainly suitable for people with blood deficiency of the liver, heart, and spleen meridians, and is mostly used for people with a thin body, palpitation, shortness of breath, spontaneous sweating, dysmenorrhea due to blood deficiency, dry stool and excessive and clear urine.

Patients with deficiency of both qi and blood as the main syndrome, mainly present palpitation, shortness of breath, fatigue, spontaneous sweating, insomnia, forgetfulness, and unwillingness to talk.

People with blood deficiency and blood stasis mainly present insomnia, dysmenorrhea, thirst with a desire to drink warm water, trance, and dark tongue.

Those with deficiency cold and abdominal pain as the main syndrome, mainly present fear of cold, fatigue, abdominal pain, reduced appetite and thin stool.

◎ *Applicable syndrome*

Danggui (Angelicae Sinensis Radix) can be used for the treatment of ischemic stroke, thromboangiitis obliterans, hypertension, iron deficiency anemia, dysmenorrhea, chronic diarrhea, etc., which belong to syndromes of qi and blood deficiency, blood deficiency with blood stasis, defcieincy cold with abdominal pain.

◎ *What kinds of people are not suitable for Danggui (Angelicae Sinensis Radix)?*

Because Danggui (Angelicae Sinensis Radix) is slightly pungent and warm, and has the function of harmonizing blood and enriching blood, it is not suitable for those who are always afraid of heat and like cold, and those who like to drink cold water due to stomach heat.

If there is fear of heat, stomach heat, and diarrhea after taking Danggui (Angelicae Sinensis Radix), stop using it, and take Huanglian (Coptidis Rhizoma) water appropriately to relieve the symptoms.

### [Diet Therapy Recommended by the Doctor]

◎ *Usage and dosage of Danggui (Angelicae Sinensis Radix) in diet therapy*

Danggui (Angelicae Sinensis Radix) is sweet, warm, and has a moderate effect. 5–15g can be used as a substitute for tea in daily life. 10–30g of decoction pieces can be used in cuisine, such as stir-frying, cooking soup, and making porridge.

◎ *What season is Danggui (Angelicae Sinensis Radix) most suitable for taking?*

Danggui (Angelicae Sinensis Radix) can be taken all year round because it has the function of enriching blood and promoting blood circulation, especially in autumn and winter.

◎ *How to combine Danggui (Angelicae Sinensis Radix) with other medicinal materials and food ingredients?*

Danggui (Angelicae Sinensis Radix) is pugent, sweet and warm. When it is used to enrich the blood and nourish deficiency, especially to boost qi and nourish blood of the heart and spleen, brown sugar or honey is often added to enhance its effect. It is often combined with Taoren (Persicae Semen), Honghua (Carthami Flos), Ejiao (Asini Corii Colla) and Aiye (Artemisiae Argyi Folium) for the treatment of blood stasis and amenorrhea, abdominal pain with a preference for pressure, cold hands and feet.

In daily cooking, it is often combined with medicinals of warming yang and dispelling cold, such as Huangqi (Astragali Radix), Rougui (Cinnamomi Cortex), and Shengjiang (Zingiberis Rhizoma Recens), to achieve the effect of warming yang and enriching blood. For congee, it can often be combined with

Taoren (Persicae Semen) and Honghua (Carthami Flos) to reduce swelling and relieve pain. For soup, it can often be combined with Renshen (Ginseng Radix et Rhizoma), Huangqi (Astragali Radix) and Rougui (Cinnamomi Cortex) to invigorate qi and nourish blood.

◎ *How to choose Danggui (Angelicae Sinensis Radix) and Huangqi (Astragali Radix) as a diet therapy?*

Danggui (Angelicae Sinensis Radix) and Huangqi (Astragali Radix) are both sweet and warm, which have the diet therapy effect of enriching blood and nourishing deficiency. They are often used together to improve the curative effect of each other. Compared with Huangqi (Astragali Radix), Danggui (Angelicae Sinensis Radix) can moisten intestines and relieve constipation. Therefore, it is more suitable for those with blood deficiency, intestine dryness, and dry stool.

**Small experiential recipe**

To treat qi and blood consumption after blood loss, or qi and blood deficiency, fatigue, and dizziness.

*Danggui (Angelicae Sinensis Radix) 10g and Huangqi (Astragali Radix) 60g are decocted in water. Drink 100ml twice a day.*

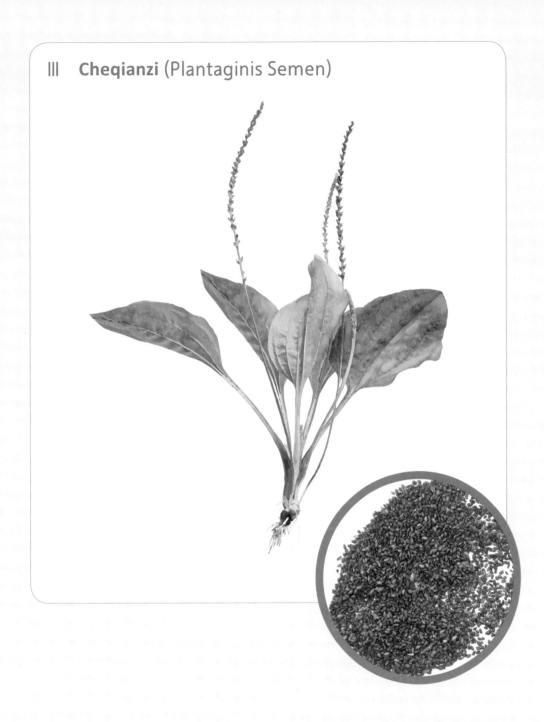

# Ⅲ **Cheqianzi** (Plantaginis Semen)

◎ *Which is better to use as medicine, big one or small one?*

Cheqianzi (Plantaginis Semen) of large size is mainly produced in southern provinces, while small one is mainly produced in North China, Northeast China, and Northwest China. They are only different in variety and have no obvious difference in quality.

◎ *How to distinguish the quality of Cheqianzi (Plantaginis Semen)?*

Large, plump and even seeds with brown-red color are of good quality.

◎ *How to preserve Cheqianzi (Plantaginis Semen)?*

Dried Cheqianzi (Plantaginis Semen) usually can be stored for a long time (about 1 year) in an airtight jar in a cool and dry place.

◎ *What is the difference among raw, dry-fried, and saltwater-fried Cheqianzi (Plantaginis Semen)?*

Cheqianzi (Plantaginis Semen) decoction pieces are divided into raw Cheqianzi (Plantaginis Semen), dry-fried Cheqianzi (Plantaginis Semen), and saltwater-fried Cheqianzi (Plantaginis Semen). Raw Cheqianzi (Plantaginis Semen) has a good diuretic effect on promoting water circulation, especially promoting urination. Dry-fried Cheqianzi (Plantaginis Semen) with its abated coldness has a good effect of eliminating dampness and relieving diarrhea. When fried with saltwater, it is mainly used to tonify the liver and kidney and improve eyesight.

[Efficacy Told by the Doctor]

◎ *Medicinal properties and efficacy—clearing heat, promoting urination, relieving diarrhea, improving eyesight, and eliminating phlegm*

Cheqianzi (Plantaginis Semen) is sweet and bland and TCM believes that bland medicinals have the effects of promoting urination and percolating dampness, and its medicinal properties is slightly cold, so it can clear heat and promote diuresis. Cheqianzi (Plantaginis Semen) enters the lung, liver, kidney, and bladder meridans to remove dampness-heat from these viscera. Therefore, it also has the functions of clearing heat, relieving diarrhea, clearing the lung, eliminating phlegm, clearing the liver and improving eyesight.

◎ *Applicable people—damp-heat constitution, poor urination, diarrhea, and dry eyes*

Cheqianzi (Plantaginis Semen) is mainly suitable for people with the damp-heat constitution, especially those with the damp-heat accumulation in the lung, liver, kidney, and bladder. It is mostly used for those who are usually afraid of heat, have dry and red eyes, cough and asthma, even cough with blood, abdominal distension, edema of limbs, poor urination, and thin stool, and women with much yellowish leucorrhea.

Patients with cough and asthma due to lung heat are mainly manifested by cough and asthma, yellow phlegm, chest pain, even hemoptysis, dry throat, vexation heat, etc.

People with red eyes due to liver fire mainly present vexation and irritability, bitter mouth and dry throat, dry eyes with redness and pain, more eye droppings, yellow urine, and so on.

Patients with damp-heat diarrhea mainly present abdominal distension, chest diaphragm discomfort after eating, diarrhea, bowel sounds, and abdominal pain.

Patients with inhibited urination due to dampness-heat mainly present edema of limbs, sluggish urination or dripping poorly, or heat and pain in urination, even hematuria, and more yellowish leucorrhea in women.

◎ *Applicable syndrome*

Cheqianzi (Plantaginis Semen) can be used for the treatment of asthma, pneumonia, diarrhea, gastrointestinal dysfunction, acute glomerulonephritis, chronic nephritis, conjunctivitis, and visual fatigue, which belong to the syndrome of dampness-heat accumulation.

◎ *What kinds of people are not suitable for Cheqianzi (Plantaginis Semen)?*

Because Cheqianzi (Plantaginis Semen) is slightly cold, it is not suitable for people who are weak in constitution, overworked, always afraid of cold and liking warmth, lack of yang, and have spermatorrhea due to kidney deficiency. TCM believes that "all seeds are descending", so the medicinal property of Cheqianzi (Plantaginis Semen) is descending, which is not suitable for people with gastroptosis, uterine prolapse, and rectocele.

If there is fear of cold, cold stomach, spermatorrhea, and efflux discharge after taking Cheqianzi (Plantaginis Semen), stop using it, and take Rougui (Cinnamomi Cortex) appropriately to relieve the symptoms.

**[Diet Therapy Recommended by the Doctor]**

◎ *Usage and dosage of Cheqianzi (Plantaginis Semen) in diet therapy*

Cheqianzi (Plantaginis Semen) is sweet, bland, and gentle in medicinal properties. 5–10g can be used as a substitute for tea in daily life. 10–15g of decoction pieces can be used for home meals such as soup and congee.

◎ *What season is Cheqianzi (Plantaginis Semen) most suitable for taking?*

Cheqianzi (Plantaginis Semen) can be taken all year round. Because it has the functions of clearing heat, promoting urination and improving eyesight, it is especially suitable for taking in summer and autumn.

◎ *How to combine Cheqianzi (Plantaginis Semen) with other medicinal materials and food ingredients?*

Cheqianzi (Plantaginis Semen) is sweet, bland and slightly cold, and it is often combined with Zhizi (Gardeniae Fructus), Xiaoji (Cirsii Herba), Maogen (Imperatae Rhizoma), etc., to clear heat and promote urination and treat hematuria due to blood heat. For the elderly benign prostatic hyperplasia or prostatitis and poor urination, it is often combined with Shengdihuang (Rehmanniae Radix), Dongkuizi (Malvae Fructus) and Shiwei (Pyrrosiae Folium). It is used to treat dry or swollen eyes, and is often combined with Juemingzi

(Cassiae Semen), Jinyinhua (Lonicerae Japonicae Flos), Gouqi (Lycii Fructus), etc., to enhance the effects of clearing the liver and improving eyesight.

It is often cooked with Yiyiren (Coicis Semen), Baibiandou (Lablab Semen Album), and Shanyao (Dioscoreae Rhizoma) as congee to clear heat, strengthen the spleen and stop diarrhea; it is often cooked with a black-bone chicken, or a duck or a carp as soup to induce diuresis to alleviate edema.

◎ *How to choose Cheqianzi (Plantaginis Semen) and Cheqiancao (Plantaginis Herba) as a diet therapy?*

Cheqianzi (Plantaginis Semen) and Cheqiancao (Plantaginis Herba) have similar functions, both of which have diet therapy effects such as clearing heat, inducing diuresis, and arresting diarrhea. However, Cheqiancao (Plantaginis Herba) also has the effects of clearing heat and detoxifying. Oral administration can treat heat-toxic sores, furuncle, blood-heat urine, damp-heat diarrhea, etc. Fresh leaves are often mashed and applied to wounds, with the effects of arresting blood, relieving inflammation, and promoting healing.

### Small experiential recipe

*1. To treat excessive leucorrhea in women*

9g of Cheqiancao (Plantaginis Herba) root is mashed and mixed with glutinous rice washing water for drinking.

*2. To treat hypertension*

30g of Cheqianzi (Plantaginis Semen) and 30g of Yuxingcao (Houttuyniae Herba) are decocted with water and taken warm.

# IV   **Sanqi** (Notoginseng Radix et Rhizoma)

◎ *Which part of the plant is used as Sanqi (Notoginseng Radix et Rhizoma)?*

The root and rhizome of Araliaceae perennial plant *Panax notoginseng* (Burk.) F. H. Chen is used as Sanqi (Notoginseng Radix et Rhizoma) in clinical practice.

◎ *How to distinguish the quality of Sanqi (Notoginseng Radix et Rhizoma)?*

Sanqi (Notoginseng Radix et Rhizoma) with dry and heavy body, large size, firm texture, smooth skin, and gray-green or gray-black color in transverse section is of good quality.

◎ *How to preserve Sanqi (Notoginseng Radix et Rhizoma)?*

Moisture will make dried Sanqi (Notoginseng Radix et Rhizoma) easy to go moldy, so the dried products should be wrapped in thick paper or cloth bags and placed in a cool and ventilated place.

[Efficacy Told by the Doctor]

◎ *Medicinal properties and efficacy—removing blood stasis and stopping bleeding, promoting blood circulation and relieving pain*

Sanqi (Notoginseng Radix et Rhizoma) is sweet, slightly bitter and warm, good at stopping bleeding, promoting blood circulation and removing blood stasis. It can be applied to all kinds of bleeding inside and outside the human body, whether there is blood stasis or not, especially for those with blood stasis. In addition, it promotes blood circulation and removes blood stasis to reduce swelling and relieve pain, which is a good choice for treating blood stasis syndromes and an important medicine for traumatology. It is the first choice for traumatic injury, tendon fracture, blood stasis, swelling and pain, etc.

◎ *Applicable population—blood stasis constitution, bruises, heart and stomach pain, exhaustion and strain*

Sanqi (Notoginseng Radix et Rhizoma) is mainly suitable for the following symptoms which belong to static blood block: hematemesis, nosebleeds, hemoptysis, hematochezia, hematuria and other internal and external bleeding; large intestine bleeding, uterine bleeding, postpartum bleeding; traumatic injury, broken tendon, fracture, swelling, pain; carbuncle, sore, heart and stomach pain.

In addition, Sanqi (Notoginseng Radix et Rhizoma) has the function of tonifying deficiency and strengthening the body, which is suitable for people with deficiency and labor injury.

◎ *Applicable syndrome*

Sanqi (Notoginseng Radix et Rhizoma) can be used for bruises, dysmenorrhea, hypertension, hepatitis, heart and stomach pain and other diseases belonging to blood stasis syndrome.

◎ *What kinds of people are not suitable for using Sanqi (Notoginseng Radix et Rhizoma)?*

Sanqi (Notoginseng Radix et Rhizoma) has the function of promoting blood circulation and removing blood stasis, so pregnant women should not use it. women with dysmenorrhea and menstrual disorder caused by deficiency of qi and blood, present dull pain in the lower abdomen with preference for pressure during menstruation or after menstruation are forbidden to take it.

**[Diet Therapy Recommended by the Doctor]**

◎ *Usage and dosage of Sanqi (Notoginseng Radix et Rhizoma) in diet therapy*

There are two ways to eat Sanqi (Notoginseng Radix et Rhizoma). Sanqi (Notoginseng Radix et Rhizoma) can be made into powder, and taken directly with boiled water, 3–5g for each time and twice a day. In addition, chicken or spareribs can be stewed with it, and the amount of Sanqi (Notoginseng Radix et Rhizoma) can be about 15g, which can invigorate qi, nourish blood, and strengthen the body, for the treatment of metrorrhagia, postpartum weakness, spontaneous sweating and night sweating. It also treats headache, weak and sour lumbar muscles of the elderly.

◎ *What season is Sanqi (Notoginseng Radix et Rhizoma) most suitable for taking?*

It can be taken all year round.

◎ *How to combine Sanqi (Notoginseng Radix et Rhizoma) with other medicinal materials and food ingredients?*

For hemoptysis, hematemesis, epistaxis, hematuria and hematochezia, Sanqi (Notoginseng Radix et Rhizoma) can be used alone, or combined with Huaruishi (Ophicalcitum) and Xueyutan (Crinis Carbonisatus). Sanqi (Notoginseng Radix et Rhizoma) stewed with chicke can tonify qi and blood, and is used for people with blood stasis due to deficiency of qi and blood. It can also be used for coronary heart disease, cerebrovascular disease and traumatic injury.

### Small experiential recipe

*1. To treat hematemesis and epistaxis*
Sanqi (Notoginseng Radix et Rhizoma) powder 5g, chew first and then swallow with rice soup.
*2. To treat female blood stranguria*
Sanqi (Notoginseng Radix et Rhizoma) powder 5g, take with Dengxincao (Junci Medulla) and ginger soup.

## V  **Maidong** (Ophiopogonis Radix)

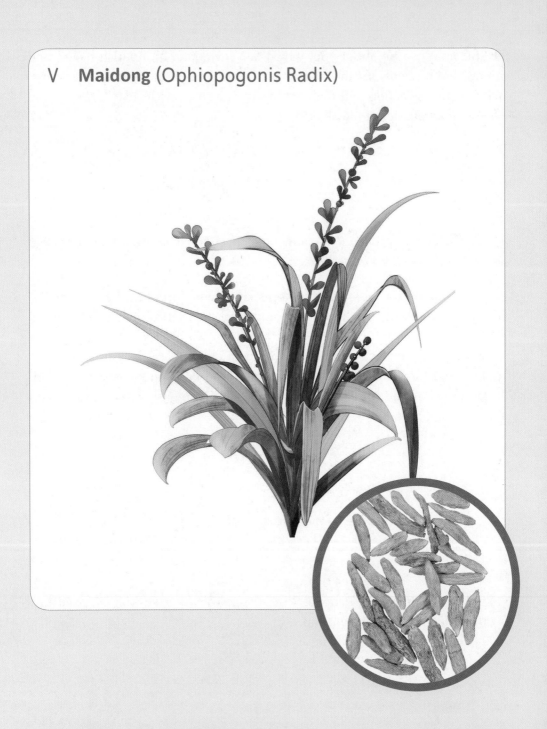

## [Drug Selection by the Pharmacist]

◎ *Which part of the plant is used as Maidong (Ophiopogonis Radix)?*

The root tuber of Liliaceae plant *Ophiopogon japonicus* (L. f.) Ker-Gawl. is used as medicine.

◎ *Where is the best Maidong (Ophiopogonis Radix) produced?*

Maidong (Ophiopogonis Radix) produced in Zhejiang has a better quality.

◎ *How to distinguish the quality of Maidong (Ophiopogonis Radix)?*

Maidong (Ophiopogonis Radix) with a yellowish-white surface, dry and big body, soft texture, translucence, aroma, and stickiness is of good quality.

◎ *How to preserve Maidong (Ophiopogonis Radix)?*

Maidong (Ophiopogonis Radix) contains several saccharides, which is easy to absorb moisture and become oily. If it needs to be stored for a long time, it should be placed in an airtight container and kept away from light. Keep it in a cool and dry place, moisture-proof.

## [Efficacy Told by the Doctor]

◎ *Medicinal properties and efficacy—nourishing yin, moistening the lung, benefiting the stomach, and clearing the heart*

Maidong (Ophiopogonis Radix) is sweet and slightly cold, which has a tonic effect. It enters the lung and stomach meridians, so it can nourish yin and moisten the lung, benefit the stomach and promote fluid production. Its taste is also slightly bitter, and it enters the heart meridian. TCM believes that bitter medicinals can clear heat, so it can clear the heart and relieve dysphoria and has a good effect of clearing the heart and tranquilizing the mind.

◎ *Applicable people—yin deficiency constitution, dry throat, chronic cough, dysphoria, and insomnia*

Maidong (Ophiopogonis Radix) is mainly suitable for people with yin deficiency and internal heat in the lung, stomach, and heart, and is mostly used for those who are thin, cannot bear heat, are prone to night sweat, have insomnia, thirst with a desire to drink cold water, dry stool, and less and yellow urine.

Patients with yin deficiency and lung dryness mainly present dry cough with less phlegm, hemoptysis, dry throat, hoarseness, dysphoria and heat, night sweat, and so on.

Patients with yin deficiency and stomach heat mainly have dry mouth and lips, gastric upset, retching, decreased intake of food, discomfort in the chest and diaphragm after eating, dry stool, and so on.

Those with deficiency heat disturbing the heart often present insomnia, palpitation, trance, emotion out of control, bitter taste, yellow urine, and so on.

◎ *Applicable syndrome*

Maidong (Ophiopogonis Radix) can be used for the treatment of tuberculosis, pneumonia, pharyngolaryngitis, congestive heart failure, chronic pulmonary heart disease, coronary atherosclerotic heart disease, viral myocarditis, chronic atrophic gastritis, diabetes, which belong to the symdromes of yin deficiency and lung dryness, yin deficiency and stomach heat, and deficiency heat disturbing the heart.

◎ *What kinds of people are not suitable for Maidong (Ophiopogonis Radix)?*

Because Maidong (Ophiopogonis Radix) is slightly cold and has the function of nourishing yin and moistening the lung, it is not suitable for people with exogenous wind-cold cough, cold intolerance, preference for warmth, a cold stomach and thin stool.

If there is fear of cold, cold stomach and diarrhea after taking Maidong (Ophiopogonis Radix), stop using it and take Shengjiang (Zingiberis Rhizoma Recens) water appropriately to relieve the symptoms.

◎ *Usage and dosage of Maidong (Ophiopogonis Radix) in diet therapy*

Maidong (Ophiopogonis Radix) is sweet and gentle, 10–15g of decoction pieces can be used as a daily substitute for tea, or for cuisine, such as soup and congee.

◎ *What season is Maidong (Ophiopogonis Radix) best for taking?*

Maidong (Ophiopogonis Radix) can be taken all year round. Because it has the functions of moistening the lung and clearing heart fire, it is especially suitable for taking in summer and autumn.

◎ *How to combine Maidong (Ophiopogonis Radix) with other medicinal materials and food ingredients?*

Maidong (Ophiopogonis Radix) is sweet, cold, and moist. For its yin-nourishing effect, especially nourishing lung yin, it is often accompanied by white sugar or honey to enhance its yin-nourishing and dryness-moistening effect. It is often combined with Tiandong (Asparagi Radix), Yuzhu (Polygonati Odorati Rhizoma), Baihe (Lilii Bulbus) and Shengdihuang (Rehmanniae Radix) to treat deficiency of lung yin, manifested by dry cough with less sputum or blood in sputum, vexing heat of palms and soles, night sweat, etc.

It is often cooked as congee with mung beans, Yiyiren (Coicis Semen), etc., to clear heat and strengthen the spleen. It can often be cooked as soup with black-bone chicken, Yuzhu (Polygonati Odorati Rhizoma) and Gouqizi (Lycii Fructus) to nourish yin and moisten dryness.

◎ *How to choose Maidong (Ophiopogonis Radix) and Shashen (Adenophorae Radix, Glehniae Radix)?*

Maidong (Ophiopogonis Radix) and Shashen (Adenophorae Radix, Glehniae Radix) are sweet and cold, which enter the lung and stomach meridians and have the diet therapy effects of clearing the lung and nourishing yin, clearing heat, and promoting fluid production. They are often used together to improve the curative effect of each other. Compared with Shashen (Adenophorae Radix,

Glehniae Radix), Maidong (Ophiopogonis Radix) can also clear the heart and tranquillize the mind, so it is more suitable for people with insomnia, palpitation, and dreaminess. In addition, Maidong (Ophiopogonis Radix) can also be used for fever, fluid consumption and intestinal dryness, and constipation. Nanshashen (Adenophorae Radix) has the function of eliminating phlegm, and it is more suitable for dry cough with sticky sputum caused by fluid consumption.

## Small experiential recipe

*1. To treat heart heat, boredom, thirst, red tongue, and less fluid*

Maidong (Ophiopogonis Radix) 15g, fresh bamboo leaves 10g, millet 100g. Decoct Maidong (Ophiopogonis Radix) and bamboo leaves to get the decoction. Add the decoction when the millet is half cooked, and then cook until the congee is finished. Take congee 100g at a time, once a day.

*2. To treat angina pectoris of coronary heart disease*

Maidong (Ophiopogonis Radix) 45g, add water and decoct into 30–40ml. Divide it into several doses and take it continuously for 3–18 months.

*3. To treat constipation due to intestinal dryness*

Maidong (Ophiopogonis Radix) 15g, Dihuang (Rehmanniae Radix) 15g, Xuanshen (Scrophulariae Radix). Decoct them with water, 1 dose per day.

# VI  **Wuweizi** (Schisandrae Chinensis Fructus)

◎ *What are the main producing areas of Wuweizi (Schisandrae Chinensis Fructus)?*

The mature fruit of Magnoliaceae plant *Schisandra chinensis* (Turcz.) Baill is used as Wuweizi (Schisandrae Chinensis Fructus). It is often called "Bei Wuweizi" which is mainly produced in Northeast China.

◎ *How to process and preserve Wuweizi (Schisandrae Chinensis Fructus)?*

It should be stored in a ventilated and dry place. It can be used raw, steamed with vinegar or honey and dried.

◎ *What are the differences in the efficacy among raw product, vinegar-processed product, and honey-processed product?*

The decoction pieces of Wuweizi (Schisandrae Chinensis Fructus) are divided into raw product, vinegar-processed product and honey-processed product. The raw product has strong effects of promoting production of fluid and quenching thirst, vinegar-processed product is excellent in astringing the lung and relieving cough, and honey-proessed product has a good effect of invigorating qi and nourishing the heart.

[Efficacy Told by the Doctor]

◎ *Medicinal properties and efficacy—astringing and consolidating, invigorating qi and promoting fluid production, tonifying the kidney, and calming the heart*

Wuweizi (Schisandra Chinensis Fructus) tastes acid and sweet, and TCM believes that acid medicinals have the effect of astringency and consolidation. Its medicinal properties are warm, and it can promote production of fluid and quench thirst. Wuweizi (Schisandra Chinensis Fructus) can enter the lung, heart and kidney meridians, and tonify the deficiency of these zang-fu viscera.

Therefore, this medicinal also has the functions of astringing the lung and relieving cough, tonifying the kidney and essence, nourishing the heart, and calming the mind. In addition, it can also relieve diarrhea, arrest sweating and enuresis.

◎ *Applicable people—qi and yin deficiency constitution, asthma due to long-term illness, spermatorrhea and night emission, chronic diarrhea, thirst due to fluid consumption*

Wuweizi (Schisandra Chinensis Fructus) is mainly suitable for people with deficiency of qi and yin, especially for patients with chronic deficiency of the lung, heart, and kidney. It is mostly used for people with deficiency of qi and yin, manifested by asthma, spontaneous sweating and night sweating, thirst due to fluid consumption, palpitation, spermatorrhea, night emission, soreness of the waist and knees, infertility, chronic diarrhea, insomnia, and dreaminess.

Patients with cough and asthma due to lung deficiency as the main symptom usually present cough caused by long-term disease, expectoration, panting, obvious wheezing after activities, fatigue, chest tightness, and so on.

Patients with fluid damage and thirst as the main symptom usually have fever, vexation, thirst with a desire to drink, but failing to resolve thirst, dry mouth and throat, and so on.

Patients with long-term diarrhea as the main symptom often present abdominal distension, poor appetite, the discomfort of the chest and diaphragm after eating, diarrhea with watery discharge or undigested food, diarrhea before dawn, and so on.

Patients with spermatorrhea and night emission as the main diseases often present soreness and weakness of the waist and knees, cold semen, impotence, premature ejaculation, infertility, and so on.

◎ *Applicable syndrome*

Wuweizi (Schisandra Chinensis Fructus) can be used to treat asthma, diarrhea, liver function damage, arrhythmia, hypertension, infertility, Alzheimer's disease, Parkinson's disease and other diseases with the syndrome of deficiency of both qi and yin.

◎ *What kinds of people are not suitable for Wuweizi (Schisandra Chinensis Fructus)?*

Because Wuweizi (Schisandra Chinensis Fructus) is slightly warm and good at astringing, it is not suitable for patients with exogenous diseases, phlegm dampness, dampness-heat, blood stasis, food accumulation, etc. Patients with an aversion to cold, fever, excessive phlegm, red tongue, thick and greasy tongue coating, yellow urine, and dry stool should use it with caution.

**[Diet Therapy Recommended by the Doctor]**

◎ *Usage and dosage of Wuweizi (Schisandra Chinensis Fructus) in diet therapy*

Wuweizi (Schisandra Chinensis Fructus) is acid, sweet, and astringent and 1–3g can be used as a daily substitute for tea.

◎ *What season is Wuweizi (Schisandra Chinensis Fructus) most suitable for taking?*

Wuweizi (Schisandra Chinensis Fructus) can be taken all year round. Because it has an astringent effect, it is especially suitable for taking in autumn and winter.

◎ *How to combine Wuweizi (Schisandra Chinensis Fructus) with other medicinal materials and food ingredients?*

Wuweizi (Schisandra Chinensis Fructus) is sweet and astringent, and can be used with Shanzhuyu (Corni Fructus), Shudihuang (Rehmanniae Radix Praeparata), Shanyao (Dioscoreae Rhizoma), and Yingsuke (Papaveris Pericarpium) when it is used to astringe lung and relieve cough for the treatment of deficient athma due to chronic diseases. It can be combined with Mahuang (Ephedrae Herba), Xixin (Asari Radix et Rhizoma), Ganjiang (Zingiberis Rhizoma), etc., to treat cough with external cold and internal fluid retention syndrome. It can be used with Huangqi (Astragali Radix), Mahuanggen (Ephedrae Radix et Rhizoma), Fuxiaomai (Tritici Levis Fructus), and Muli (Ostreae Concha) when treating spontaneous sweating and night sweating. It tonifies the kidney, astringes spermatorrhea and prevents enuresis, and is a common medicine for treating spermatorrhea and night emission due to kidney deficiency, so it can be used with Sangpiaoxiao (Mantidis Oötheca), Longgu (Draconis Os), Tusizi (Cuscutae Semen), Fupenzi (Rubi Fructus), Shanzhuyu (Corni Fructus), Shudihuang (Rehmanniae Radix Praeparata), and Shanyao (Dioscoreae Rhizoma). It can be used with Wuzhuyu (Euodiae Fructus), Buguzhi (Psoraleae Fructus), and Roudoukou (Myristicae Semen) to treat chronic diarrhea due to spleen and kidney deficiency and cold. It is often used with Renshen (Ginseng Radix et Rhizoma), Maidong (Ophiopogonis Radix), Shanyao (Dioscoreae Rhizoma), Zhimu (Anemarrhenae Rhizoma), and Tianhuafen (Trichosanthis Radix) to treat profuse sweating and thirst due to heat impairing qi and yin.

It can often be cooked as congee with Qianshi (Euryales Semen), Baibiandou (Lablab Semen Album), and Shanyao (Dioscoreae Rhizoma) to strengthen the spleen and tonify the kidney. It is also cooked as soup with black-bone chicken, soft-shelled turtle, and sea cucumber to tonify the kidney and and strengthen essence.

◎ *How to choose Bei Wuweizi (Schisandrae Chinensis Fructus) and Nan Wuweizi (Schisandrae Sphenantherae Fructus) as a diet therapy?*

There is little difference in efficacy between Bei Wuweizi and Nan Wuweizi, and both can be used as a substitute for tea. Bei Wuweizi has a good effect on tonifying the kidney and is suitable for kidney deficiency, manifested by spermatorrhea, night emission, soreness of waist and knees, impotence, premature ejaculation, and infertility.

**Small experiential recipe**

*1. To treat insomnia and forgetfulness*
One perch, Wuweizi (Schisandrae Chinensis Fructus) 50g, appropriate amount of cooking wine, refined salt, scallion segments, ginger slices, pepper powder, and oil. Soak Wuweizi (Schisandra Chinensis Fructus) and wash it clean. Remove the scales, gills, and viscera from the perch, wash and put it into a casserole, then add appropriate amount of cooking wine, salt, scallion segments, ginger slices, raw oil, clear water, and Wuweizi (Schisandra Chinensis Fructus); cook until the fish is pureed; remove onion and ginger, and season with pepper powder. Once a week, several times a

day with no restriction.

*2. To treat hyposexuality and frequent nocturia*

Tusizi (Cuscutae Semen) 100g, Wuweizi (Schisandrae Chinensis Fructus) 50g, a low-alcohol liquor 100ml. Wash and dry Tusizi (Cuscutae Semen) in the sun, put them into a wine bottle, seal after adding wine, shake once a day, soak for 10 days, and then start drinking. 2 times a day, 15ml each time.

*3. To treat chronic illness and cough due to deficiency*

Wuweizi (Schisandrae Chinensis Fructus) 250g. Add appropriate amount of water, boil it to obtain decoction, concentrate into a watery paste, add the same amount or a proper amount of honey, decoct over low fire, and wait until it cools down. 1–2 teaspoonful each time, take with boiled water on an empty stomach.

# VII Luhui (Aloe)

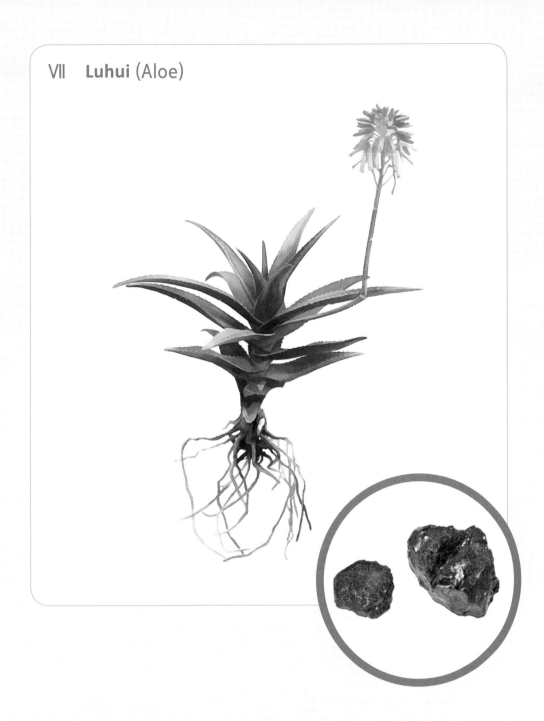

◎ *Which part of the plant is used as Luhui (Aloe)?*

The sap concentrate of the Liliaceae plant leaves of *Aloe barbadensis* Miller, *Aloe ferox* Miller, or other related plants of the same genus.

◎ *What are the main producing areas of Luhui (Aloe)?*

As early as Tang Dynasty, Luhui (Aloe) was introduced into China from Iran. Nowadays, *Aloe vera* L. var. *chinensis* (Haw.) Berg. is a unique variety in China, mainly cultivated in Fujian, Taiwan, Guangdong, Guangxi, Sichuan, and Yunnan.

◎ *How to store Luhui (Aloe)?*

Store in a cool and ventilated place away from light.

◎ *Medicinal properties and efficacy—clearing the liver and purging fire, purging constipation, killing worms, and treating malnutrition*

Luhui (Aloe) is bitter and cold and enters the liver and large intestine meridians. Cold can remove heat, bitter can dry dampness and purge heat, and can also kill worms. It enters the liver meridian, purges the excessive fire of the liver meridian, and treats constipation, dizziness, headache, and irritability. It enters the large intestine meridian, purges and relieves constipation, and is used for constipation due to heat.

◎ *Applicable people—exuberant liver fire*

Luhui (Aloe) is more suitable for people with a strong constitution (called excess pattern in TCM). Peolple with hypertension and constipation, energetic people, and people with red faces, or who easily lose temper all belong to this category.

The main clinical manifestations of patients with exuberant liver fire are dizziness, severe distending pain, red face and eyes, bitter mouth, dry mouth, irritability, tinnitus, short yellow urine, constipation, red tongue and yellow tongue coating, wiry and rapid pulse.

◎ *Applicable syndrome*

Luhui (Aloe) is mainly suitable for people with constipation due to heat accumulation, headache, red eyes, convulsion, abdominal pain due to parasite accumulation, scabies, hemorrhoids and other diseases belonging to hyperactive liver fire.

◎ *What kinds of people are not suitable for Luhui (Aloe)?*

Luhui (Aloe) is bitter and cold. Pharmacological studies have proved that Luhui (Aloe) contains anthraquinone derivatives such as aloe emodin, which will produce adverse reactions in the digestive tract after decomposition in vivo, so pregnant women and children with deficiency cold of the spleen and stomach are forbidden to take it.

**[Diet Therapy Recommended by the Doctor]**

◎ *Diet therapy usage and dosage of Luhui (Aloe)*

Oral administration: in the form of pill and powder, 0.5–1.5g.

External use: Appropriate amount, grind it and apply on the affected area. As a vegetable, the conventional dosage of fresh aloe vera is about 15g per day.

◎ *What season is Luhui (Aloe) most suitable for taking?*

Luhui (Aloe) can be taken all year round. Intake of Luhui (Aloe) in summer can reduce the body's absorption of fatty oil in food and achieve the purpose of weight loss and detoxification.

◎ *How to combine Luhui (Aloe) with other medicinal materials and food ingredients?*

Luhui (Aloe) is often used with Longdan (Gentianae Radix et Rhizoma),

Huangqin (Scutellariae Radix), Huangbo (Phellodendri Chinensis Cortex), Huanglian (Coptidis Rhizoma), Dahuang (Rhei Radix et Rhizoma), and Danggui (Angelicae Sinensis Radix) to treat mania, irritability, fright, and convulsion caused by the excessive fire in liver meridian. For the treatment of abdominal pain due to roundworm, it can be combined with Shijunzi (Quisqualis Fructus) and Kulianpi (Meliae Cortex). Fresh aloe vera can be eaten raw as cold dish, and juiced, but the elderly, children, and people who are allergic to it should not eat it.

◎ *How to choose Luhui (Aloe) and Fanxieye (Sennae Folium) as a diet therapy?*

Luhui (Aloe) and Fanxieye (Sennae Folium) can purge and relieve constipation and are good at treating constipation due to heat accumulation, but Luhui (Aloe) is good at clearing liver heat and can be used for infantile malnutrition. Fanxieye (Sennae Folium) is good at purging and removing stagnation and can eliminate swelling and move water and treat ascites swelling.

### Small experiential recipe

*1. To treat constipation*

Before going to bed every night, 5g of fresh aloe vera leaves and 30g of honey are infused with boiling water to relieve constipation.

*2. To treat infantile malnutrition*

Equal amount of Shijunzi (Quisqualis Fructus) and aloe vera leaves. Dry them in the sun, grind them into fine powder, and mix them with rice soup, 3–6g each time.

*3. To treat scalds*

Wash appropriate fresh aloe vera leaves according to the burn area, peel off epidermis, apply the gel to the disinfected burn site, and then cover and fix it with disinfectant gauze. Change the dressing every 1–3 hours on the same day, and 2–3 times a day later. Generally, the pain can be relieved or disappear within 1–3 hours, and the redness and swelling gradually subside. It heals in 2–8 days with no scars left.

# VIII  **Shihu** (Dendrobii Caulis)

◎ *Which part of the plant is used as Shihu (Dendrobii Caulis)?*

The medicinal parts are mainly fresh or dry stems.

◎ *What are the main producing areas of Shihu (Dendrobii Caulis)?*

Shihu (Dendrobii Caulis) is cultivated in most provinces south of the Yangtze River, especially in Anhui, Zhejiang, Yunnan, Guizhou, Guangdong and Guangxi.

◎ *How to store Shihu (Dendrobii Caulis)?*

Shihu (Dendrobii Caulis) is often stored at room temperature (not to exceed 20°C). When stored, it should be placed in a dry and ventilated place at home. Avoid direct exposure to the sun. It can also be stored in the fresh-keeping layer of the refrigerator at 3–5 °C for cold storage, which can be stored for 3–6 months.

**[Efficacy Told by the Doctor]**

◎ *Medicinal properties and efficacy—benefiting stomach, promoting fluid production, nourishing yin, and clearing heat*

Shihu (Dendrobii Caulis) can nourish. With its slightly cold and cool nature, it is used for clearing and nourishing. It enters the stomach meridian and can nourish stomach yin and produce body fluid; it enters the kidney meridian and can nourish kidney yin and clear deficiency heat. It is suitable for thirst, dry lips, or excessive fluid consumption after heatstroke, dry mouth, red tongue, low fever, and so on.

◎ *Applicable people—excessive heat damaging fluid and insufficient stomach yin*

Shihu (Dendrobii Caulis) is mainly used for people with excessive heat and deficiency of stomach yin.

Patients with excessive heat damaging fluid mainly present yellow tongue coating, fever, and thirst with a desire to drink.

Patients with deficiency of stomach yin mainly present fullness, vomiting, and hiccup, accompanied by dry mouth, dry throat, red tongue with little tongue coating, and thin and fast pulse.

◎ *Applicable syndrome*

Shihu (Dendrobii Caulis) can be used to treat chronic pharyngitis, thromboangiitis obliterans, arthritis, skin suppurative infection, and other diseases.

◎ *What kinds of people are not suitable for Shihu (Dendrobii Caulis)?*

Shihu (Dendrobii Caulis) has the effects of benefiting stomach, promoting fluid production, nourishing yin and clearing heat, so those with yang deficiency and cold, warm febrile diseases, and damp-warm not transforming into dryness are forbidden to take it. Otherwise it may aggravate the illness in severe cases. Pregnant women should also follow the doctor's advice to avoid overdose.

**[Diet Therapy Recommended by the Doctor]**

◎ *Usage and dosage of Shihu (Dendrobii Caulis) in diet therapy*

The dosage of Shihu (Dendrobii Caulis) is generally 6–12g; while 15–30g for the fresh products. Excessive consumption of Shihu (Dendrobii Caulis) can cause harm to the human body. Therefore, the dosage of Shihu (Dendrobii Caulis) for healthy and subhealthy people should be controlled within 3–5g, while 10–20g for the fresh products.

◎ *What season is Shihu (Dendrobii Caulis) most suitable for taking?*

Tiepishihu (Dendrobii Caulis) is most suitable for taking in winter. Every year from December to February, it is the harvest season of Shihu (Dendrobii Caulis). At this time, Shihu (Dendrobii Caulis) has the highest nutritional and medicinal value. Shihu (Dendrobii Caulis) has the effect of nourishing yin and promoting fluid production. In winter, the temperature is low, and the weather is dry. Shihu (Dendrobii Caulis) can help nourish viscera and relieve dryness.

◎ *How to combine Shihu (Dendrobii Caulis) with other medicinal materials and food ingredients?*

Shihu (Dendrobii Caulis) combined with Tianhuafen (Trichosanthis Radix), or Maidong (Ophiopogonis Radix), Nanshashen (Adenophorae Radix), Shanyao (Dioscoreae Rhizoma), and Yuzhu (Polygonati Odorati Rhizoma) can be used to treat people with deficiency cold in the stomach. When eaten together with Nanshashen (Adenophorae Radix), Pipaye (Eriobotryae Folium), Shengdihuang (Rehmanniae Radix), Maidong (Ophiopogonis Radix), Baihe (Lilii Bulbus), Qinjiao (Gentianae Macrophyllae Radix), Yinchaihu (Stellariae Radix) and Rendongteng (Lonicerae Japonicae Caulis), it can treat symptoms such as deficiency heat, dry mouth and abnormal sweating due to general debility.

Shihu (Dendrobii Caulis), Dongchongxiacao (Cordyceps), water duck, etc., cooked as soup can nourish stomach yin, nourish kidney yin, moisten the lung, and tonify the spleen. With pork, Shengjiang (Zingiberis Rhizoma Recens), Maidong (Ophiopogonis Radix), etc., it can clear stomach heat, promote production of fluid, quench thirst, nourish the kidney, bring down fever and improve eyesight.

◎ *How to choose Shihu (Dendrobii Caulis) and Yuzhu (Polygonati Odorati Rhizoma) as a diet therapy?*

Shihu (Dendrobii Caulis) and Yuzhu (Polygonati Odorati Rhizoma) can nourish yin, but Yuzhu (Polygonati Odorati Rhizoma) tastes sweet and is juicy and has the effects of tonifying deficiency, clearing heat, promoting production of fluid and quenching thirst. Shihu (Dendrobii Caulis) can nourish yin and clear heat, nourish the stomach and fortify the spleen, stop polydipsia and reduce stomach fire, which achieves the effects of clearing and tonifying the middle.

---

**Small experiential recipe**

*To treat hypertension of liver-fire flaming upward type*

Shihu (Dendrobii Caulis) 15g (decocted first), Shijueming (Haliotidis Concha) 30g (decocted first), Sangjisheng (Taxilli Herba) 15g, Juemingzi (Cassiae Semen) 10g. The above ingredients are decocted in water. One dose a day and taken two times a day.

# IX Honghua (Carthami Flos)

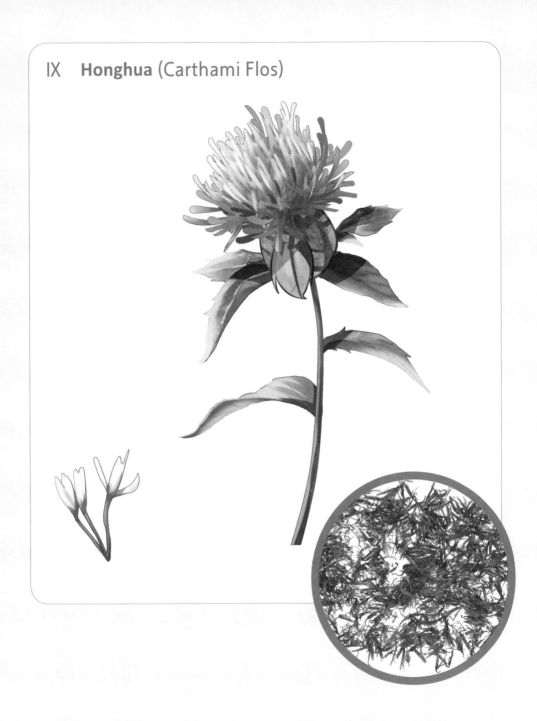

◎ *Which part of the plant is used as Honghua (Carthami Flos)?*

Dried flowers of Compositae plant *Carthamus tinctorius* L. is used as medicine.

◎ *What are the main producing areas of Honghua (Carthami Flos)?*

Honghua (Carthami Flos) originated in Iran, Spain, and other countries. In addition, it has been introduced and cultivated in Henan, Jiangsu, Shanghai, and other provinces or cities in China. Now the largest producing area of Honghua (Carthami Flos) in China is Xinjiang.

◎ *How to store Honghua (Carthami Flos)?*

Honghua (Carthami Flos) should be placed in a cool and dry place, moisture-proof and moth-proof. If dampness is found, open the container to dry or dry over a mild fire in time, and then pack and seal it for preservation after the hot air diffuses and cools down thoroughly. Be careful not to expose it to the sun.

◎ *How to choose Honghua (Carthami Flos) with good quality?*

The surface is red-yellow or red, the color is bright, and the stamen is cylindrical which is slightly forked on top. It feels soft and has a slightly bitter taste. When it is soaked in the water, the water turns orange-red with a light fragrance. The above are characteristics of good quality.

[Efficacy Told by the Doctor]

◎ *Medicinal properties and efficacy—promoting blood circulation, dispersing blood stasis, dredging meridians, and relieving pain*

Honghua (Carthami Flos) is warm in nature and pungent in taste; it belongs to liver and heart meridians. It can move blood, disperse blood stasis and relieve pain. It is red, bitter, and warm, and it goes into the blood phase of the heart and liver. It is a medicinal characterized by dissipating; it can invigorate blood when used in a small dosage, while used in a large dosage, it can promote blood circulation. Therefore, it is good at treating blood stasis.

◎ *Applicable people—blood stasis constitution, irregular menstruation*

Honghua (Carthami Flos) can be used to treat dysmenorrhea, amenorrhea, and postpartum abdominal pain and is also suitable for various blood stasis symptoms, traumatic injury, coronary heart disease, and other diseases. People who have blood stasis in the body can take it under the guidance of a doctor.

People with a blood stasis constitution often have a dark face, purple tongue or petechia, thin white or thin yellow tongue coating, choppy or wiry pulse; less menstruation with dark color and blood clots in women.

◎ *Applicable syndrome*

Honghua (Carthami Flos) can be used to treat trauma, occlusive cerebrovascular disease, coronary heart disease, myocardial infarction, vasculitis, and other diseases. It also has an adjuvant therapeutic effect on hyperlipidemia, diabetic complications, irregular menstruation, rheumatoid arthritis, and so on.

◎ *What kinds of people are not suitable for using Honghua (Carthami Flos)?*

Honghua (Carthami Flos) is not suitable for people with coagulation dysfunction and bleeding tendency. Usually, women with more menstruation or pregnancy should also use it with caution.

**[Diet Therapy Recommended by the Doctor]**

◎ *Usage and dosage of Honghua (Carthami Flos) in diet therapy*

Oral administration of Honghua (Carthami Flos): 3–10g for decoction, 3–5g for nourishing and invigorating blood when soaked in water and used as a drink, and 6–10g for promoting blood circulation and removing blood stasis, instead of tea.

◎ *What season is Honghua (Carthami Flos) most suitable for taking?*

It can be eaten all year round.

◎ *How to combine Honghua (Carthami Flos) with other medicinal materials and food ingredients?*

Honghua (Carthami Flos) with Taoren (Persicae Semen): Honghua (Carthami Flos) can promote blood circulation and remove blood stasis, dredge meridians and relieve pain because its pungent flavor has the function of dissipation and its warm nature has the function of unblocking; Taoren (Persicae Semen) is sweet and bitter, which can moisten and descend. Its nature is not biased. It has the functions of promoting blood circulation, removing blood stasis and moistening the intestines to promote defecation. The two medicinals are combined to bring out the best in each other, and to enhance the effects of promoting blood circulation and removing blood stasis. So it is applicable to any pattern of blood stasis.

Soaking Honghua (Carthami Flos) with Dazao (Jujubae Fructus), Taoren (Persicae Semen), Danggui (Angelicae Sinensis Radix) and Chenpi (Citri Reticulatae Pericarpium) in water can effectively improve the symptoms of pale complexion, burnout and fatigue caused by deficiency of qi and blood, as well as women's less menstruation with pale color; replacing tea with Shengjiang (Zingiberis Rhizoma Recens), Baishao (Paeoniae Radix Alba), Fengmi (Mel) and Sangye (Mori Folium) can relieve joint pain, back pain and other symptoms caused by blood stasis blocking meridians.

◎ *How to choose Honghua (Carthami Flos) and Zanghonghua (Croci Stigma) as a diet therapy?*

Zanghonghua (Croci Stigma) is a kind of precious Chinese herbal medicine. Although their names are similar, their effects are different. Zanghonghua (Croci Stigma) has the effects of promoting blood circulation and removing blood stasis, cooling blood, detoxifying, and tranquillizing. It can treat amenorrhea, postpartum blood stasis, depression, fright and delirium, and other related symptoms. Honghua (Carthami Flos) has the effects of promoting blood circulation, dredging meridians, reducing swelling, and relieving pain. Still, its blood circulation function is not as strong as Zanghonghua (Croci Stigma).

*1. To treat dysmenorrhea*

Honghua (Carthami Flos) 6g, Jixueteng (Spatholobi Caulis) 30g. Decoct with water to get juice, add a proper amount of yellow wine, and take it at one time.

*2. To treat arthritis swelling and pain*

After frying Honghua (Carthami Flos), grind it into powder, add the same amount of sweet potato powder, mix it with salt water or Chinese liquor, and apply it to the affected part.

# X   Tianma (Gastrodiae Rhizoma)

◎ *Which part of the plant is used as Tianma (Gastrodiae Rhizoma)?*

The dried tuber of Orchidaceae plant *Gastrodia elata* Bl. is used as medicine.

◎ *Where is the best Tianma (Gastrodiae Rhizoma) produced?*

Tianma (Gastrodiae Rhizoma) produced in Zhaotong, Yunnan Province has the best quality.

◎ *How to distinguish the quality of Tianma (Gastrodiae Rhizoma)?*

It is better to be horn-like, translucent in tansverse section and yellow and white in color.

◎ *How to preserve Tianma (Gastrodiae Rhizoma)?*

Fresh Tianma (Gastrodiae Rhizoma) can be gently washed with water, dried in the sun, sealed with newspapers and plastic bags, and put into the refrigerator for cold storage. The newly dug Tianma (Gastrodiae Rhizoma) cannot be scratched. Put it into a box, cover it with a layer of sand and with a film, do not seal it, and store it in a dry place at about 10°C. Dried Tianma (Gastrodiae Rhizoma) should be put in a glass, sealed and stored in a cool and ventilated place. It can not be frozen, or it is easy to deteriorate.

◎ *What is the difference between Tianma (Gastrodiae Rhizoma) produced in winter and that produced in spring?*

Tianma (Gastrodiae Rhizoma) is mainly divided into winter Tianma (Gastrodiae Rhizoma) and spring Tianma (Gastrodiae Rhizoma). Winter Tianma (Gastrodiae Rhizoma) has a full appearance with few wrinkles, yellow and white color, is not easy to break and has a better quality. Spring Tianma (Gastrodiae Rhizoma) has thick wrinkles with gray and brown color, and it is easy to break and poor in quality.

◎ *Medicinal properties and efficacy—relieving wind and spasm, stabilizing liver yang, dispelling wind, and dredging collaterals*

Tianma (Gastrodiae Rhizoma) is sweet and not biased. It belongs to the liver meridian, and has the functions of relieving wind and spasm, stabilizing liver yang, dispelling wind, and dredging collaterals. It is good at relieving wind and spasm, and treats a variety of liver wind diseases, including both internal wind and external wind. It can also stabilize liver yang and treat hyperactivity of liver yang.

◎ *Applicable people—invasion of external wind, internal movement of liver wind and hyperactivity of liver yang*

Tianma (Gastrodiae Rhizoma) mainly treats people with internal movement of liver wind and hyperactivity of liver yang. It is mostly used for headaches, dizziness, wind pathogen, limb spasm, and infantile convulsion.

Those who catch external wind mainly present rheumatic arthralgia, sluggish joint movement, pain in bones and muscles, etc.

Those who have internal movement of liver wind mainly present vertigo, convulsion, and convulsion in children.

Patients with hyperactivity of liver yang mainly present headache, dizziness, red face and red eyes, impatience, irritability, vexation, and insomnia.

◎ *Applicable syndrome*

Tianma (Gastrodiae Rhizoma) can be used for hypertension, vertigo, convulsions, rheumatic pain, insomnia and other diseases belonging to liver yang hyperactivity.

◎ *What kinds of people are not suitable for Tianma (Gastrodiae Rhizoma)?*

Patients with blood and yin deficiency, fluid loss and low blood pressure should use it with caution.

# [Diet Therapy Recommended by the Doctor]

◎ *Usage and dosage of Tianma (Gastrodiae Rhizoma) in diet therapy*

Tianma (Gastrodiae Rhizoma) tastes sweet and is not biased, so, as s diet therapy, it can be used for steaming, boiling, and stewing with other ingredients, and the daily dosage should not exceed 40g.

◎ *What season is Tianma (Gastrodiae Rhizoma) most suitable for taking?*

Tianma (Gastrodiae Rhizoma) can be taken all year round. Because of its strong nourishing property, it is better to be taken in winter.

◎ *How to combine Tianma (Gastrodiae Rhizoma) with other medicinal materials and food ingredients?*

It can be combined with Jiangcan (Bombyx Batryticatus), Quanxie (Scorpio), and Gouteng (Uncariae Ramulus cum Uncis) when treating acute infantile convulsion. Combined with Jiangcan (Bombyx Batryticatus), Renshen (Ginseng Radix et Rhizoma) and Baizhu (Atractylodis Macrocephalae Rhizoma), it can treat chronic infantile convulsion due to spleen defiency. Combined with Zhitiannanxing (Arisaematis Rhizoma Preparatum), Quanxie (Scorpio) and Jiangcan (Bombyx Batryticatus), it is used to treat infantile convulsions of various types. It can be used in combination with Fangfeng (Saposhnikoviae Radix), Tiannanxing (Arisaematis Rhizoma) and Baifuzi (Typhonii Rhizoma) to treat opisthotonus and tetanus. It treats dizziness caused by hyperactivity of liver yang with Shijueming (Haliotidis Concha), Gouteng (Uncariae Ramulus cum Uncis) and Niuxi (Achyranthis Bidentatae Radix). It is often compatible with Qinjiao (Gentianae Macrophyllae Radix), Qianghuo (Notopterygii Rhizoma et Radix), Sangzhi (Mori Ramulus), Moyao (Myrrha), Zhiwutou (Aconiti Kusnezoffii Radix Cocta, prepared), etc., to treat numbness and dysfunction of hands and feet caused by stroke.

In daily cooking, combined with pork and pig brain, it can nourish the brain; as congee it is cooked together with japonica rice and pig brain to calm the liver and calm the wind, promote qi and blood circulation.

*To treat dizziness*

Tianma (Gastrodiae Rhizoma) 30g, 3 eggs, 1,000ml of water. Boil eggs with Tianma (Gastrodiae Rhizoma) in the water, and then eat eggs.

# XI Dihuang (Rehmanniae Radix)

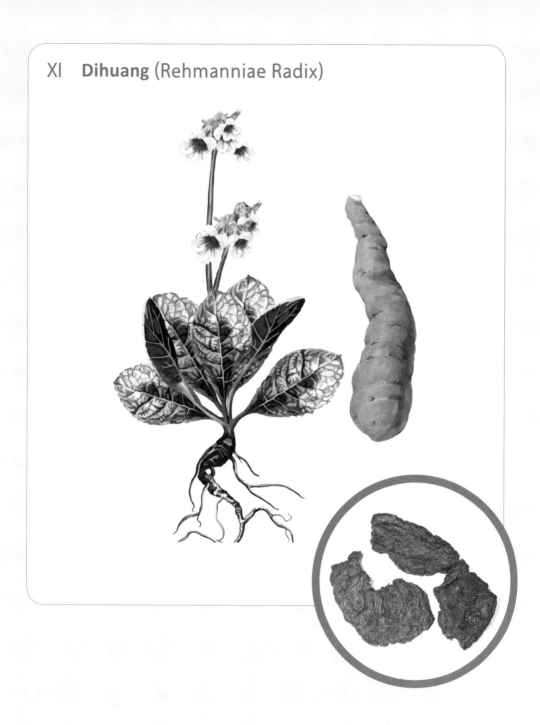

◎ *Which part of the plant is used as Dihuang (Rehmannia Glutinosa)?*

The fresh or dried root tuber of Scrophulariaceae plant *Rehmannia glutinosa* Libosch. is used as medicine.

◎ *Where is the best Dihuang (Rehmanniae Radix) produced?*

The quality of Dihuang (Rehmanniae Radix) produced in Henan is the best.

◎ *How to distinguish the quality of Dihuang (Rehmanniae Radix)?*

Dihuang (Rehmanniae Radix) can be divided into Shengdihuang (Rehmanniae Radix) and Shudihuang (Rehmanniae Radix Praeparata) according to different processing methods. Shengdihuang (Rehmanniae Radix) is regarded to have a good quality if its transverse section is pitch black, while Shudihuang (Rehmanniae Radix Praeparata) is regarded to have a good quality if its transverse section is pitch black and its taste is sweet.

◎ *How to preserve Dihuang (Rehmanniae Radix)?*

Shudihuang (Rehmanniae Radix Praeparata) can be sealed and stored in a dry and cool place to prevent deterioration from air and water. It can also be sealed and frozen in the refrigerator to prolong the storage time. Shengdihuang (Rehmanniae Radix) can be sliced, dried, sealed and stored in a dry cool place or refrigerated.

◎ *What is the difference between Shengdihuang (Rehmanniae Radix) and Shudihuang (Rehmanniae Radix Praeparata)?*

Decoction pieces of Dihuang (Rehmanniae Radix) are often divided into two types: Shengdihuang (Rehmanniae Radix) and Shudihuang (Rehmanniae Radix Praeparata). Shengdihuang (Rehmanniae Radix) is obtained by removing the reed head, fibrous root, and silt from Xiandihuang (Rehmanniae Radix Recens) and is baked until about 80% dry. Shudihuang (Rehmanniae Radix Praeparata) is prepared by stewing Shengdihuang (Rehmanniae Radix) with wine until the wine is sucked up, air-drying until the mucus on the surface is slightly dry, cutting into pieces or thick slices, and drying for later use. Shengdihuang

(Rehmanniae Radix) is sweet and cold, mainly for clearing heat and cooling blood, nourishing yin and promoting fluid production, while Shudihuang (Rehmanniae Radix Praeparata) is sweet and slightly warm, mainly for enriching blood and nourishing yin, benefiting essence and supplementing marrow.

## [Efficacy Told by the Doctor]

◎ *Medicinal properties and efficacy—Shengdihuang (Rehmanniae Radix): clearing heat and cooling blood, nourishing yin, and promoting fluid production; Shudihuang (Rehmanniae Radix Praeparata): enriching the blood, nourishing yin, benifiting essence and supplementing marrow*

Shengdihuang (Rehmanniae Radix) tastes sweet, and is cold in nature. It belongs to the heart, liver, and kidney meridians. It enters the nutrient and blood levels, and is good at clearing heat and cooling blood. It is mostly used to treat ecchymoses, unconsciousness, delirium, etc., caused by warm diseases with heat entering the nutrient and blood levels. It can also treat bleeding due to blood heat. Because of its cold nature, sweet taste, and moisture texture, it can nourish yin and promote fluid production, and treat yin deficiency diseases such as polydipsia and bone steaming, and tidal fever.

Shudihuang (Rehmanniae Radix Praeparata) tastes sweet, is mildly warm, and belongs to liver and kidney meridians. With the main effects of enriching blood and nourishing yin, it is good at benefiting essence and supplementing marrow. It is an important medicine for treating blood deficiency, and is mainly used for liver and kidney yin deficiency syndrome.

◎ *Applicable people—Shengdihuang (Rehmanniae Radix): heat entering the nutrient and blood levels, blood-heat bleeding, yin deficiency, and fever; Shudihuang (Rehmanniae Radix Praeparata): various syndromes of blood deficiency and deficiency of liver and kidney*

Shengdihuang (Rehmanniae Radix) is suitable for patients with heat entering the blood, bleeding, and yin injury.

Patients with heat entering the nutrient and blood levels mainly present high fever, polydipsia, unconsciousness, crimson tongue, petechiae or ecchymoses, rashes, delirium, and so on.

Patients with blood heat hemorrhage mainly present hematemesis, epistaxis, hematochezia, metrorrhagia, metrostaxis, hematuria, postpartum hemorrhage, and so on.

Patients with yin deficiency and fever mainly present vexation, thirst, excessive drinking, and tidal fever after bone steaming, night fever and abating at dawn, intestinal dryness, and constipation.

**Shudihuang (Rehmanniae Radix Praeparata)** is suitable for people with deficiency of yin and blood and insuficiency of the liver and kidney.

Sallow complexion, palpitation, insomnia, dizziness, metrorrhagia, metrostaxis and irregular menstruation can be seen in those with blood deficiency.

For patients with deficiency of the liver and kidney present soreness of waist and knees, tinnitus, deafness, spermatorrhea, night sweat, wasting thirst, tidal fever after bone steaming, prematurely white hair and beard, five retardations (retardation of standing, walking, speaking, hair and teeth growing) and five kinds of infantile flaccidity (soft head, mouth, hands, feet, and muscles) can be seen.

◎ *Applicable syndrome*

Sheng Dihuang (Rehmanniae Radix) can be used to treat blood-heat bleeding, bone steaming and hot flashes belonging to yin deficiency and blood heat syndrome; Shudihuang (Rehmanniae Radix Praeparata) can be used to treat osteoporosis, palpitation, insomnia and tinnitus, which belong to liver and kidney deficiency syndrome.

◎ *What kinds of people are not suitable for Dihuang (Rehmanniae Radix)?*

Because Shengdihuang (Rehmanniae Radix) is cold, it is not suitable for people with spleen deficiency and dampness or a full abdomen and loose stool. Shudihuang (Rehmanniae Radix Praeparata) is greasy, obstructs the stomach, and is difficult to digest, so patients with excessive dampness, stagnant qi, excessive phlegm, and abdominal fullness are forbidden to take it. If it must be taken, it can be combined with Sharen (Amomi Fructus) and Chenpi (Citri

Reticulatae Pericarpium).

## [Diet Therapy Recommended by the Doctor]

◎ *Usage and dosage of Dihuang (Rehmanniae Radix) in diet therapy*

10–30g of Dihuang (Rehmanniae Radix) every day is suitable for making soup, congee, and stewing meat.

◎ *What season is Dihuang (Rehmanniae Radix) most suitable for taking?*

It can be taken all year round. Because Dihuang (Rehmanniae Radix) is sweet and moist, it is suitable for nourishing yin. "Nourishing yang in spring and summer, nourishing yin in autumn and winter", so it is more suitable to take in autumn and winter.

◎ *How to combine Dihuang (Rehmanniae Radix) with other medicinal materials and food ingredients?*

Shengdihuang (Rehmanniae Radix) tastes sweet and is cold in nature and can be combined with Lianqiao (Forsythiae Fructus), Xuanshen (Scrophulariae Radix), and Huanglian (Coptidis Rhizoma) to treat high fever, unconsciousness, vexation, thirst and crimson tongue. Combined with Chishao (Paeoniae Radix Rubra), Mudanpi (Moutan Cortex), and Shuiniujiao (Bubali Cornu), it can treat ecchymoses, unconsciousness and delirium. Combined with Daqingye (Isatidis Folium) and Shuiniujiao (Bubali Cornu), it can be used to treat excessive heat toxin, ecchymoses and rashes in dark purple color. Combined with Cebaiye (Platycladi Cacumen), Diyu (Sanguisorbae Radix), Huaihua (Sophorae Flos), Xiaoji (Cirsii Herba) and Qiancao (Rubiae Radix et Rhizoma), it treats hemorrhage. It is compatible with Shashen (Adenophorae Radix, Glehniae Radix) and Maidong (Ophiopogonis Radix) to treat vexation, thirst and multiple drink. It is combined with Digupi (Lycii Cortex), Zhimu (Anemarrhenae Rhizoma), Maidong (Ophiopogonis Radix), Qinghao (Artemisiae Annuae Herba) and Biejia (Trionycis Carapax) to treat bone steaming and tidal fever, and night fever abating at dawn.

Shudihuang (Rehmanniae Radix Praeparata) is moist and mildly warm, and can be combined with Baishao (Paeoniae Radix Alba), Danggui (Angelicae Sinensis Radix) and Chuanxiong (Chuanxiong Rhizoma) to treat blood deficiency. It is combined with Shanzhuyu (Corni Fructus), Shanyao (Dioscoreae Rhizoma), Zhimu (Anemarrhenae Rhizoma), etc., to treat liver and kidney yin deficiency. It is combined with Heshouwu (Polygoni Multiflori Radix) and Niuxi (Achyranthis Bidentatae Radix) to treat prematurely white hair. Combined with Gouji (Cibotii Rhizoma), Suoyang (Cynomorii Herba), Guijia (Testudinis Carapax Et Plastrum), etc., it can be used to treat five retardations and five types of infantile flaccidity.

In daily life, Shengdihuang (Rehmanniae Radix) can be combined with Gouqizi (Lycii Fructus) and black-bone chicken to nourish yin and promote fluid production, and treat night sweats and backache. With lean pork, Baihe (Lilii Bulbus) and other ingredients to make soup, it nourishes the heart and relieves annoyance, calms the heart and tranquilizes the mind. Shudihuang (Rehmanniae Radix Praeparata) can also be stewed with chicken to nourish qi and blood, or stewed with mutton as soup to help yang rise.

## Small experiential recipe

**1. To treat soreness of waist and knees and tinnitus**

Shudihuang (Rehmanniae Radix Praeparata) 50g, 1 pig's trotter, Duzhong (Eucommiae Cortex) 30g, Gouqizi (Lycii Fructus) 30g, Niuxi (Achyranthis Bidentatae Radix) 30g. The above ingredients are stewed and eaten at meal time.

**2. To treat dry cough, dry throat, thirst, etc.**

Shudihuang (Rehmanniae Radix Praeparata) 40g, enucleated Dazao (Jujubae Fructus) 6 pieces, Dongchongxiacao (Cordyceps) 10g, duck 500g. Put the first three into the belly of the old duck, add water, stew for 3 hours over a mild fire, and eat at meal time.

**3. To treat uterine bleeding**

Shengdihuang (Rehmanniae Radix) 30g, Danggui (Angelicae Sinensis Radix) 30g, mutton 250g, a proper amount of salt. Stew for soup.

**4. To treat butterfly spots**

Shengdihuang (Rehmanniae Radix) 100g, Gouqizi (Lycii Fructus) 30g, Shanyao (Dioscoreae Rhizoma) 200g, white duck 500g. Marinate white duck with scallions, ginger, and condiment, and steam them with the above ingredients and eat at meal time.

# Section 3
## Precious Chinese Medicinals

| **Renshen** (Ginseng Radix et Rhizoma)

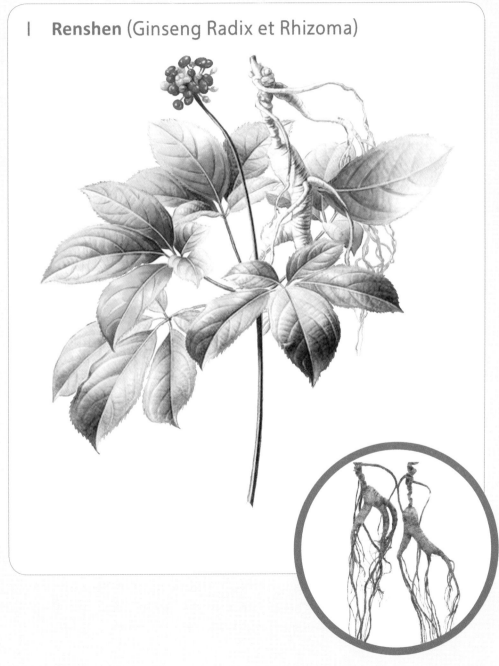

◎ *Which part of the plant is used as Renshen (Ginseng Radix et Rhizoma)?*

The root and rhizome of Araliaceae plant *Panax ginseng* C. A. Mey. is used as medicine.

◎ *Where is the best Renshen (Ginseng Radix et Rhizoma) produced?*

Renshen (Ginseng Radix et Rhizoma) in Fusong County, Jilin Province, has the largest yield and the best quality, which is called Jilin Renshen (Ginseng Radix et Rhizoma).

◎ *What do the various names of Renshen (Ginseng Radix et Rhizoma) mean?*

Wild Renshen (Ginseng Radix et Rhizoma) is named "Shanshen". Cultivated ginseng is called "Yuanshen", Which should be cultivated for 6–7 years and harvested.

Fresh ginseng washed and dried and is called "Shengshaishen". Fresh ginseng steamed and dried is called "Hongshen". The fine roots collected when ginseng is processed are called "Shenxu (ginseng whiskers)". Shanshen is called "Shengshai Shanshen (sun-dried mountain ginseng)" after being dried in the sun.

◎ *How to choose Shanshen?*

Shanshen with large body, long reeds, spiritual body, fine skin and bright yellow color, fine grain and full lines, and no injuries is of good quality.

◎ *In terms of application, what are the differences among Shanshen, Hongshen, Shengshaishen and Shenxu?*

Shanshen is a great supplement to vitality, which is the best product of Renshen (Ginseng Radix et Rhizoma). Hongshen is vigorous, warm, and dry, and has the effect of invigorating qi, especially inspiring yang. Shengshaishen is mild and suitable for strengthening body resistance and eliminating pathogenic factors. The effect of Shenxu is small and moderate.

◎ *Medicinal properties and efficacy—tonifying vitality, invigorating the spleen and kidney, promoting fluid production, and tranquilizing the mind*

Renshen (Ginseng Radix et Rhizoma) is sweet and slightly warm, and can replenish primordial qi, and return yang qi from extinction. It is the first important medicine for treating internal injuries caused by asthenia. Therefore, Renshen (Ginseng Radix et Rhizoma) alone is very effective for original qi loss or collapse with manifestations such as massive blood loss, profuse sweating, severe vomiting and diarrhea. Renshen (Ginseng Radix et Rhizoma) entering the spleen meridian can tonify the spleen, regulate the spleen and stomach, invigorate the spleen qi, help transport body fluid to achieve the effect of promoting production of fluid and quenching thirst. In addition, as Renshen (Ginseng Radix et Rhizoma) strongly supplement original qi, it can calm the mind because sufficient qi nourishes the mind.

◎ *Applicable people—collapse of original qi, deficiency of lung and spleen qi, and febrile diseases damaging the fluid*

Renshen (Ginseng Radix et Rhizoma) is mainly suitable for people with deficiency of original qi and fluid damage due to qi deficiency. It is mostly used for people with deficiency of qi and blood after blood loss and ulceration, manifested by pale complexion, aversion to cold and fever, cold hands and feet, spontaneous sweating or cold sweating, and fine and weak pulse.

Those who mainly have collapse of original qi commonly have a pale face, shortness of breath, fatigued limbs, dizziness, cold hands and feet, and fine and weak pulse.

Patients with deficiency of lung and spleen qi mainly present loss of appetite, thin stool, listlessness, emaciation, fatigued limbs, weak breath and unwillingness to talk, spontaneous sweating and fear of wind, susceptibility to external pathogen, sallow or white complexion, or edema of limbs, pale tongue with white tongue coating, slow and weak pulse, etc.

Patients with febrile diseases damaging fluid mainly present tiredness and fatigue, listlessness, palpitation, shortness of breath, dry cough, less phlegm, dry throat and crimson tongue, thirst and drinking a lot, dry stool, and so on.

◎ *Applicable syndrome*

Renshen (Ginseng Radix et Rhizoma) can be used for the treatment of critically ill people with almost collapse of original qi, manifested by shortness of breath, lassitude, and weak pulse verging on expiry caused by profuse sweating, severe diarrhea, massive blood loss, severe or long-term illness, or people with weak spleen and stomach and loss of appetite, or people with thirst, fatigue, hyperhidrosis and weak pulse in the later stage of febrile diseases.

◎ *What kinds of people are not suitable for Renshen (Ginseng Radix et Rhizoma)?*

Because Renshen (Ginseng Radix et Rhizoma) is a kind of qi-invigorating medicine, people should not take it casually if there is no signs of qi deficiency. Especially for people with a strong constitution, it is not prope to take tonics if there is no weakness. Irrational use of Renshen (Ginseng Radix et Rhizoma) such as misuse or multi-use, often leads to suspended breathing, chest tightness, and abdominal distension.

In addition, avoid eating radishes and drinking tea after taking Renshen (Ginseng Radix et Rhizoma).

**[Diet Therapy Recommended by the Doctor]**

◎ *Usage and dosage of Renshen (Ginseng Radix et Rhizoma) in diet therapy*

Renshen (Ginseng Radix et Rhizoma) is sweet, warm, and slightly bitter, and 5–15g can be used as a substitute for tea in daily life. 10–20g of decoction pieces can be used for home meals such as stew, soup, and porridge.

◎ *What season is Renshen (Ginseng Radix et Rhizoma) most suitable for taking?*

Renshen (Ginseng Radix et Rhizoma) is sweet, warm, and slightly bitter, so we must pay attention to seasonal changes when taking it. Generally speaking, it is better to be taken in autumn and winter when the weather is cool.

◎ *How to combine Renshen (Ginseng Radix et Rhizoma) with other medicinal materials and food ingredients?*

Renshen (Ginseng Radix et Rhizoma) can replenish original qi, restore the pulse, and relieve desertion, and it is effective to be used alone, such as "Dushen Decoction". If qi deficiency causes desertion and is accompanied by sweating, and cold limbs, it should be used together with Fuzi (Aconiti Lateralis Radix Praeparata) to invigorate qi for relieving desertion. If qi deficiency causes desertion and is accompanied by sweating, and warm body, thirst with a preference for cold drinks, and a red and dry tongue, it is often combined with Maidong (Ophiopogonis Radix) and Wuweizi (Schisandrae Chinensis Fructus) to invigorate qi, nourish yin and astringe sweat. As for spleen deficiency failing to transport, it is often used with Baizhu (Atractylodis Macrocephalae Rhizoma), Fuling (Poria), Huangqi (Astragali Radix), and Danggui (Angelicae Sinensis Radix). If heat damages qi and fluid, it is often used with Zhimu (Anemarrhenae Rhizoma) and Shigao (Gypsum Fibrosum).

In daily stewing and soup cooking, it is often matched with japonica rice, lean meat, chickens, ducks, fish, and other ingredients to nourish and strengthen the body.

◎ *How to choose Renshen (Ginseng Radix et Rhizoma) and Xiyangshen (Panacis Quinquefolii Radix) as a diet therapy?*

Renshen (Ginseng Radix et Rhizoma) and Xiyangshen (Panacis Quinquefolii Radix) have the effect of invigorating qi, but Renshen (Ginseng Radix et Rhizoma) has a better effect of invigorating qi than Xiyangshen (Panacis Quinquefolii Radix). Xiyangshen (Panacis Quinquefolii Radix) is cold in nature and has the functions of invigorating qi and nourishing yin, purging fire and relieving dysphoria, nourishing the stomach, and promoting fluid production. Therefore, Renshen (Ginseng Radix et Rhizoma) is more suitable for people with qi deficiency, while Xiyangshen (Panacis Quinquefolii Radix) is most suitable for people who have qi and yin deficiency with heat.

*1. To treat loss of appetite, spontaneous sweating and susceptibility to external pathogens*

Renshen (Ginseng Radix et Rhizoma) 10g, japonica rice 100g, cooked as congee. Take it warm, once in the morning and once in the evening.

*2. To treat fatigue, polydipsia and profuse drinking*

Renshen (Ginseng Radix et Rhizoma) 6g, an egg. Renshen is ground into powder, mixed well with egg white and steamed. Take it once a day.

*3. To treat sallow complexion and uneasiness*

Renshen (Ginseng Radix et Rhizoma) 5g, tremella 15g. Cook them as soup over mild fire, drink soup and eat tremella, two times a day, once in the morning and once in the evening.

## ll **Xiyangshen** (Panacis Quinquefolii Radix)

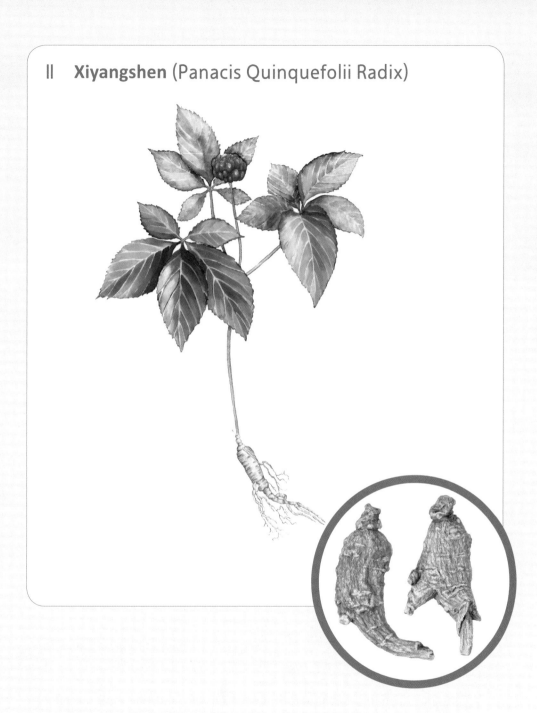

◎ *Which part of the plant is used as Xiyangshen (Panacis Quinquefolii Radix)?*

The dried root of Araliaceae plant *Panax quinquefolium* L. is used as medicine.

◎ *Where is the best Xiyangshen (Panacis Quinquefolii Radix) produced?*

Xiyangshen (Panacis Quinquefolii Radix) is usually divided into American ginseng and Canadian ginseng according to its producing area. Although they are of the same species, because of the climatic influence, the former has more obvious cross striation on surface than the latter, and more effective components.

◎ *How to distinguish the quality of Xiyangshen (Panacis Quinquefolii Radix)?*

The main root of high-quality Xiyangshen (Panacis Quinquefolii Radix) is short, mostly spindle-shaped, cylindrical or conical, often bifurcated, and the bifurcation angle is large. It has fine cross striation on surface, light weight, and less powder. It has stronge fragrance, and slightly sweet and bitter taste. The taste is refreshing and can stay for a long time. Generally, wild Xiyangshen (Panacis Quinquefolii Radix) is the top quality, followed by the cultivated one.

◎ *How to preserve Xiyangshen (Panacis Quinquefolii Radix)?*

Put the selected Xiyangshen (Panacis Quinquefolii Radix) in a certain container, store in a ventilated place, dry it, and turn it over from time to time until it dries.

◎ *What is the difference between Xiyangshen (Panacis Quinquefolii Radix) and Renshen (Ginseng Radix et Rhizoma)?*

Xiyangshen (Panacis Quinquefolii Radix) is cold and has multiple effects, such as invigorating qi and nourishing yin, purging fire and relieving dysphoria, nourishing the stomach and promoting fluid production, etc. It is mostly used for cough due to lung heat, qi deficiency and unwillingness to talk, tiredness of limbs, irritability, and loss of yin and body fluid after febrile disease. Renshen (Ginseng Radix et Rhizoma) is warm in medicinal properties, which can powerfully supplement original qi, and its tonifying power is stronger than that of Xiyangshen (Panacis Quinquefolii Radix), so it is not suitable for those who has deficiency heat due to labor. In addition, Renshen (Ginseng Radix et Rhizoma) can tonify qi of the heart and kidney, tranquillize the mind, and inprove brain function, and is also commonly used for insomnia, forgetfulness, palpitation, and shortness of breath due to failure of the kidney to receive qi.

### [Efficacy Told by the Doctor]

◎ *Medicinal properties and efficacy—invigorating qi and nourishing yin, clearing fire and promoting fluid production*

Xiyangshen (Panacis Quinquefolii Radix) tonifies original qi and nourishes yin and can tonify qi and yin of the heart, lung, and spleen. Xiyangshen (Panacis Quinquefolii Radix) is cool in nature and can clear fire and promote fluid production. It is suitable for people with hot and sweaty body, thirst, vexation, tiredness, weak breathing, weak and rapid pulse caused by heat injuring qi and fluid.

◎ *Applicable people—deficiency of both qi and yin, internal heat and fluid injury*

Xiyangshen (Panacis Quinquefolii Radix) is mainly suitable for people with deficiency of both qi and yin, internal  heat and fluid injury and is mainly used for people with damage to both qi and yin, which is mostly manifested by fever or profuse sweating, diarrhea, exhaustion, shortness of breath, spontaneous perspiration, stickiness, vexation and thirst, short and red urine, dry stool, dry tongue, thready and weak pulse.

Patients with deficiency of heart qi and yin mainly present insomnia, dreaminess, palpitation, and heartache.

Patients with deficiency of lung qi and yin mainly present shortness of breath, asthma, cough with less phlegm, or blood in phlegm.

Patients with deficiency of spleen qi and yin mainly present appetite loss, and thirst with a derie to drink.

◎ *Applicable syndrome*

Xiyangshen (Panacis Quinquefolii Radix) can be used for mental fatigue, weakness, palpitations, insomnia, cough, panting and other diseases belonging to qi and yin deficiency.

◎ *What kinds of people are not suitable for Xiyangshen (Panacis Quinquefolii Radix)?*

People with deficiency cold of the spleen and stomach are not suitable for Xiyangshen (Panacis Quinquefolii Radix). After taking Xiyangshen (Panacis Quinquefolii Radix), they will generally have fear of cold, hypothermia, loss of appetite, abdominal pain, and diarrhea; some women will have dysmenorrhea and delayed menstruation.

## [Diet Therapy Recommended by the Doctor]

◎ *Usage and dosage of Xiyangshen (Panacis Quinquefolii Radix) in diet therapy*

Xiyangshen (Panacis Quinquefolii Radix) is suitable for use as a tonic because of its mild nature. In cuisine, 3g for boiling, 2–5g for stewing, 5g for steaming, and 3–5g for infusing.

◎ *What season is Xiyangshen (Panacis Quinquefolii Radix) most suitable for taking?*

Xiyangshen (Panacis Quinquefolii Radix) can be taken all year round. Xiyangshen (Panacis Quinquefolii Radix) is a kind of "cool" ginseng, which is very suitable for "clearing and tonifying" in summer because of its effects of invigorating qi, nourishing yin, clearing fire, and promoting fluid production.

◎ *How to combine Xiyangshen (Panacis Quinquefolii Radix) with other medicinal materials and food ingredients?*

Xiyangshen (Panacis Quinquefolii Radix) in combination with Maidong (Ophiopogonis Radix): Xiyangshen (Panacis Quinquefolii Radix) benefits qi, nourishes yin, and promotes fluid production, while Maidong (Ophiopogonis Radix) enhances yin and fluid production. The two medicinals is often combined to replace tea. It is used for damage to both qi and yin due to febrile disease, dysphoria, and thirst; it is also used for older people with deficiency of qi and yin, dry throat and mouth, insufficient body fluid, dry tongue, and less tongue coating.

It is often cooked as soup with black-bone chicken, Baihe (Lilii Bulbus), Gouqizi (Lycii Fructus), and other ingredients for nourishing yin, clearing heat, and promoting fluid production, to achieve the effect of clearing heat and nourishing yin. It is combined with Chuanbeimu (Fritillariae Cirrhosae Bulbus), pear and rock sugar for yin deficiency and lung heat, cough with sticky phlegm, dry throat, and thirst.

◎ *How to choose Xiyangshen (Panacis Quinquefolii Radix) and Renshen (Ginseng Radix et Rhizoma) as a diet therapy?*

Renshen (Ginseng Radix et Rhizoma) and Xiyangshen (Panacis Quinquefolii Radix) belong to tonic medicinals. There is no essential difference in their chemical composition, and they have many physiological activities such as strengthening the body, resisting fatigue, lowering blood glucose, stabilizing the spirit, enhancing immunity, etc. Attention should be paid to different treatments in diet therapy and medicated diet. People who are with a yang heat constitution and prone to "excessive internal heat" should choose Xiyangshen (Panacis Quinquefolii Radix), while those with cold intolerance and weakness should choose sun-dried Renshen (Ginseng Radix et Rhizoma).

**Small experiential recipe**

*1. To enhance immune function*
Xiyangshen (Panacis Quinquefolii Radix) 3g (cut into slices), boil as a substitute tea and take it frequenlty.
*2. To treat persistent cough*
Xiyangshen (Panacis Quinquefolii Radix) 5g, Baihe (Lilii Bulbus) 30g, Fengmi (Mel) 80g. Steam them and eat it.
*3. To promote brain development and enhance memory*
Xiyangshen (Panacis Quinquefolii Radix) 5g, Lingzhi (Ganoderma)10g. Decoct with water, and take it twice a day.

# III Lurong (Cervi Cornu Pantotrichum)

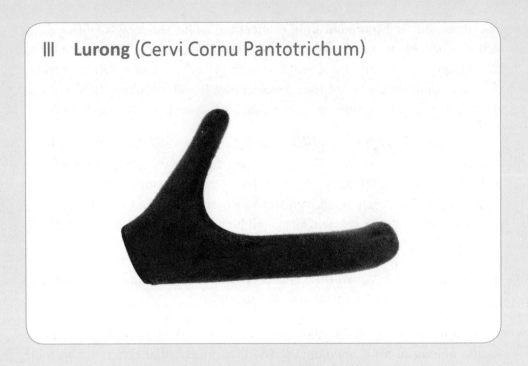

## [Drug Selection by the Pharmacist]

◎ *Which part of the anminal is used as Lurong (Cervi Cornu Pantotrichum)?*

The unossified, hairy young horns on the heads of *Cervus nippon* Temminck or *Cervus elaphus* L. are used as medicine.

◎ *How to choose Lurong (Cervi Cornu Pantotrichum)?*

Lurong (Cervi Cornu Pantotrichum): It is better to have full, round, tender, fine hair, red-brown skin, light body, and no edges at the bottom. The ones with slender, thin, rough hair, and heavy body is regarded as inferior goods.

Lurong (Cervi Cornu Pantotrichum) slices: It is better to have tender and fine pores and small red slices.

◎ *How to preserve Lurong (Cervi Cornu Pantotrichum)?*

Lurong (Cervi Cornu Pantotrichum) should be stored in a ventilated, cool and dry place, sealed. Some Sichuan pepper should be wrapped in cloth as its "protector" to preotect from insects.

## [Efficacy Told by the Doctor]

◎ *Medicinal properties and efficacy—tonifying kidney yang, benefiting essence and blood, strengthening bones and muscles, regulating Chong and Ren, and expressing sore toxins*

Lurong (Cervi Cornu Pantotrichum) is sweet and warm to tonify yang, sweet and salty to nourish the kidney, and has the nature of pure yang, so it can tonify kidney yang and benefit essence and blood. It enters the liver and kidney meridians; the kidney governs the bones, and the bones and muscles are healthy when the kidney qi is sufficient, so Lurong (Cervi Cornu Pantotrichum) also has the function of strengthening the bones and muscles. TCM believes that when the liver and kidney are sufficient, Chong and Ren can be regulated, abundant qi and blood can warm and tonify, as well as express toxin from inside, so Lurong (Cervi Cornu Pantotrichum) can regulate Chong and Ren and express sore toxin.

◎ *Applicable people—deficiency cold constitution, intolerance of cold, cold limbs, infertility due to cold uterus, five delays, and five infantile flaccidity*

Lurong (Cervi Cornu Pantotrichum) is mainly suitable for people with a deficiency cold constitution, especially those with kidney yang deficiency, kidney deficiency and weak bone, and deficiency cold of Chong and Ren. It is mostly used for intolerance of cold, impotence, premature ejaculation, infertility due to cold uterus, frequent urination, soreness of the waist and knees, dizziness and tinnitus, mental fatigue, etc.

Patients with kidney yang deficiency and decline mainly have soreness and weakness of waist and knees, intolerance of cold and cold limbs, impotence, diarrhea before dawn, listlessness, wheezing when moving, difficulty urinating or frequent nocturia, deep and weak pulse.

Patients with kidney deficiency and weak bones mainly have muscle flaccidity, spontaneous sweating when moving, night sweating when sleeping, restless sleep, five delays, or chicken breast and turtle back, thin and white tongue coating, weak and fast pulse, etc.

Patients with deficiency cold of Chong and Ren mainly have uterine deficiency cold, metrorrhagia and metrostaxis, leukorrhagia, postpartum anemia, and infertility due to cold uterus.

◎ *Applicable syndrome*

Lurong (Cervi Cornu Pantotrichum) is mainly used for kidney yang deficiency and essence and blood deficiency; flaccidity of bones and muscles due tot deficiency of liver and kidney; in gynecology, deficiency cold of Chong and Ren, and insecure Dai; long-term ulceration of sores and ulcers without healing, clear and thin pus or inward collapse of yin gangrene, and so on.

◎ *What kinds of people are not suitable for Lurong (Cervi Cornu Pantotrichum)?*

Because Lurong (Cervi Cornu Pantotrichum) is sweet, salty, and warm in nature, people who are physically strong do not need to take it or who overeat it tend to have head swelling, chest tightness or epistaxis. For the case, stop taking it immediately for observation instead of continuing to use it.

Lurong (Cervi Cornu Pantotrichum) should not be taken in the following four situations: a. People with symptoms of dysphoria with feverish sensation in chest, palms and soles and yin deficiency; b. people whose urine color is yellow and red, have dry throat or dry pain, feel polydipsia from time to time and have internal heat symptoms; c. people who often have nosebleeds, or women who have a large amount of menstruation with bright red blood, red tongue, and thin pulse, and show blood heat; d. people who catch a cold have a headache, stuffy nose, fever, chills, cough, and phlegm, dominated by external pathogen.

---

**[Diet Therapy Recommended by the Doctor]**

---

◎ *Usage and dosage of Lurong (Cervi Cornu Pantotrichum) in diet therapy*

The dosage of daily stewing is 1–4g, and that of direct mastication is 0.5–

1g. In cuisine, it is better to cook soup, or ground to make congee, or soak in wine.

◎ *What season is Lurong (Cervi Cornu Pantotrichum) most suitable for taking?*

Lurong (Cervi Cornu Pantotrichum), hot, warm, and dry, tonifies kidney yang, benefits essence and blood, and strengthens bones and muscles, so it is especially suitable to take in winter.

◎ *How to combine Lurong (Cervi Cornu Pantotrichum) with other medicinal materials and food ingredients?*

It can be used alone to tonify kidney yang, benefits essence and blood, and treat kidney yang deficiency, deficiency of essence and blood, manifested by cold limbs, impotence, premature ejaculation, infertility due to cold uterus, and frequent urination. To treat impotence, it can be soaked in wine together with Shanyao (Dioscoreae Rhizoma). It can be taken with Danggui Wumei Paste as a pill for treating exhaustion of essence and blood, dark complexion, deafness and blindness. It can be used with Renshen (Ginseng Radix et Rhizoma), Huangqi (Astragali Radix) and Danggui (Angelicae Sinensis Radix) to treat all kinds of deficiency, five kinds of strain and seven damages.

It can often be cooked with chickens or ducks, Dazao (Jujubae Fructus), Gouqizi (Lycii Fructus), Lianzi (Nelumbinis Semen), Baihe (Lilii Bulbus), Danggui (Angelicae Sinensis Radix) and Renshen (Ginseng Radix et Rhizoma); Lurong (Cervi Cornu Pantotrichum) can be soaked in white liquor for sealed storage and take 10ml every day after half a month's soakage.

◎ *How to choose Lurong (Cervi Cornu Pantotrichum) slices and Lurong (Cervi Cornu Pantotrichum) powder as a diet therapy?*

Lurong (Cervi Cornu Pantotrichum) slices and powder have the same function, and they are all processed products of Lurong (Cervi Cornu Pantotrichum). Both of them have the effects of tonifying kidney yang, benefiting essence and blood, strengthening bones and muscles, regulating Chong and Ren, and expressing sore toxins. However, the administration methods of the two are slightly different. The slices are mostly used for soaking wine, stewing, cooking soup, or chewing after cooking; while powder is suitable for congee.

*1. To treat impotence, spermatorrhea, frequent urination, soreness, and weakness of the waist and knees*

Lurong wine: Lurong (Cervi Cornu Pantotrichum) 10g, Shanyao (Dioscoreae Rhizoma)30g. Soak the two medicinals with 500g of Chinese liquor. 10–20ml at a time.

*2. To treat deficiency of essence and blood, excessive nocturia, and cold hands and feet*

Steamed eggs with Lurong: Lurong (Cervi Cornu Pantotrichum) 0.5g, ground into a fine powder, 2 eggs. Crack the eggs, pour them into a bowl, add Lurong (Cervi Cornu Pantotrichum), salt, and ground pepper, mix them well, and steam until well cooked.

*3. To treat infertility due to cold uterus*

Lurong porridge: Cook Lurong (Cervi Cornu Pantotrichum) slices (powder) and japonica rice (or millet) as porridge for eating. 0.3g of Lurong (Cervi Cornu Pantotrichum) is the appropriate amount every time.

# IV　Dongchongxiacao (Cordyceps)

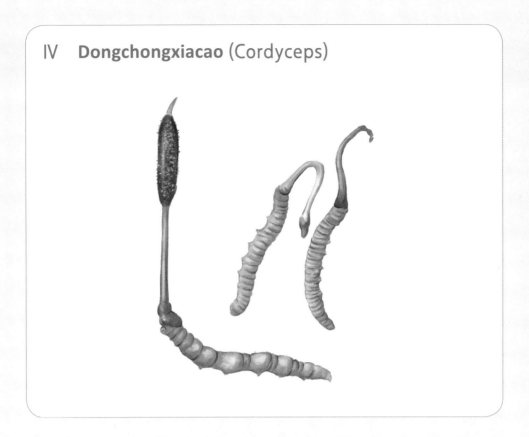

[Drug selection by the Pharmacist]

◎ *Is Dongchongxiacao (Cordyceps) a worm or grass?*

Dongchongxiacao (Cordyceps) is neither an insect nor grass, but a fungus (ascomycetes), which is a dry composite of *Cordyceps sinensis* Berk. Sacc. and bat moth larvae formed under special conditions. In winter, it appears as the body of larvae; in summer, "grass" grows from the body of larvae. So it is called "Dongchongxiacao".

◎ *Where is the best Dongchongxiacao (Cordyceps) produced?*

Dongchongxiacao (Cordyceps) mainly grows in Yushu and Guoluo in Qinghai, Naqu, Changdu, and Nyingchi in Tibet, Ganzi in Sichuan, and Diqing in Yunnan. It is generally believed that Dongchongxiacao (Cordyceps) produced in Yushu and Naqu are the best.

◎ *How to distinguish the quality of Dongchongxiacao (Cordyceps)?*

The body of Dongchongxiacao (Cordyceps) is like silkworm, with a length of about 3–5cm. It is better to have complete plump worm body, bright yellow outside, white inside, and short stroma. When Dongchongxiacao (Cordyceps) is soaked in boiling water, the body becomes enlarged and soft, and the color of the stroma becomes dark brown. The body and stroma are closely connected and do not fall off. The immersion liquid is slightly smelly. It can also be broken apart for a closer look. If there are foreign bodies such as iron wire inserted into Dongchongxiacao (Cordyceps), they are fake cordyceps.

◎ *How to preserve Dongchongxiacao (Cordyceps)?*

The newly bought Dongchongxiacao (Cordyceps) is somewhat damp and easy to be moldy and bitten by insects if left unattended for a long time. Special attention should be paid to moisture-proof, moth-proof, and insect-proof storage of Dongchongxiacao (Cordyceps). If it is in small quantity and with short storage time, it only needs to be stored in a cool and dry place. If it is in large quantity and needs to be kept for a long time, it is best to put some desiccant, such as silica gel, in the place where Dongchongxiacao (Cordyceps) is stored.

◎ *How should Dongchongxiacao (Cordyceps) be used?*

Used for general healthcare, the whole Dongchongxiacao (Cordyceps) can be soaked in water as tea to drink and then chewed. It can be crushed and taken in capsules, and can also be stewed with old ducks, or steamed with pork, or used to make Dongchongxiacao (Cordyceps) wine.

**[Efficacy Told by the Doctor]**

◎ *Medicinal properties and efficacy—sweet and not biased, tonifying the kidney, supplementing the lung, stopping bleeding and dissolving phlegm*

Dongchongxiacao (Cordyceps) is sweet in taste and not biased, which can benefit the kidney and supplement the lung, stop bleeding and dissolve phlegm. It is a very placid and precious medicine for tonifying yin and yang of the human body. It has a good tonic effect on kidney deficiency, lung qi deficiency, or lung and kidney deficiency in TCM, and its medicinal properties are mild, so it is not easy to present dryness and heat after long-term oral administration.

◎ *Applicable people—qi deficiency and yang deficiency constitution, fatigue, low back pain, spermatorrhea, chronic cough and wheezing, cough with bloody phlegm*

Dongchongxiacao (Cordyceps) is suitable for lung qi deficiency or kidney yang deficiency people, and is commonly used for weak constitution, kidney deficiency, low back pain, impotence, spermatorrhea, chronic cough and wheezing, labored cough with bloody phlegm, etc.

People with lung qi deficiency are prone to colds, and have intolerance to cold, spontaneous sweating, dry cough with less phlegm or with no phlegm, weakness, and shortness of breath.

Patients with kidney deficiency mainly have waist and knees weakness, impotence, spermatorrhea, premature ejaculation, tinnitus, forgetfulness, trance, and wheezing and cough due to kidney failing to contain qi as a result of kidney deficiency.

◎ *Applicable syndrome*

Dongchongxiacao (Cordyceps) is considered as a good medicinal for treating various deficiency diseases and can be used for respiratory diseases, cardiovascular and cerebrovascular diseases, liver cirrhosis, liver fibrosis Because it is not biased and has moderate medicinal property and can tonify yin and yang, it is also a tonic food for the elderly, the weak, the sick, and those who are still weak after childbirth. It can be taken all year round, and it is more effective to take in winter.

◎ *What kinds of people are not suitable for Dongchongxiacao (Cordyceps)?*

Although Dongchongxiacao (Cordyceps) is a top-grade tonic, it is not suitable for everyone. Generally speaking, it is suitable for patients with a deficiency constitution. If they have a strong constitution at ordinary times or have an exogenous fever, excessive dampness-heat, acute cough, or serious damage to kidney function, it is not suitable for them to continue taking it.

◎ *Usage and dosage of Dongchongxiacao (Cordyceps) in diet therapy*

Dongchongxiacao (Cordyceps) is sweet and gentle in medicinal properties, so it can be used alone but only 2g for serving each time, ground into powder, and taken on an empty stomach. 3–5g for a daily substitute for tea. Dongchongxiacao (Cordyceps) 5g can also be decocted with Duzhong (Eucommiae Cortex), Xuduan (Dipsaci Radix), etc.

In cuisine, 5–8g for soup.

◎ *What season is Dongchongxiacao (Cordyceps) most suitable for taking?*

Dongchongxiacao (Cordyceps) can be taken all year round. Because it has the function of tonifying the kidney and benefiting the lung, it is especially suitable for taking in winter.

◎ *How to combine Dongchongxiacao (Cordyceps) with other medicinal materials and food ingredients?*

Dongchongxiacao (Cordyceps) tastes sweet and is not biased. It has the effect of benefiting the lung, so, it is often stewed with Baihe (Lilii Bulbus), Chuanbeimu (Fritillariae Cirrhosae Bulbus), and tremella to treat patients with tuberculosis, manifested by cough and asthma, and bloodshot sputum. For its kidney-tonifying effect, it can be combined with Gouji (Cibotii Rhizoma), Sangjisheng (Taxilli Herba), Duzhong (Eucommiae Cortex), Xuduan (Dipsaci Radix), etc., to treat kidney deficiency, soreness and weakness of waist and knees.

In daily life, Dongchongxiacao (Cordyceps) is often stewed with chickens, ducks, beef, mutton, or various vegetables or decocted with water for the treatment of various diseases of deficiency and strain.

*1. To treat weak body, intolerance to cold and spontaneous sweating*

Dongchongxiacao (Cordyceps) 5g, an old drake, and a little yellow rice wine. Cook until well done and eat.

*2. To treat menopausal syndrome*

Dongchongxiacao (Cordyceps) 5g, a hen. Stew as soup.

# V  Lingzhi (Ganoderma)

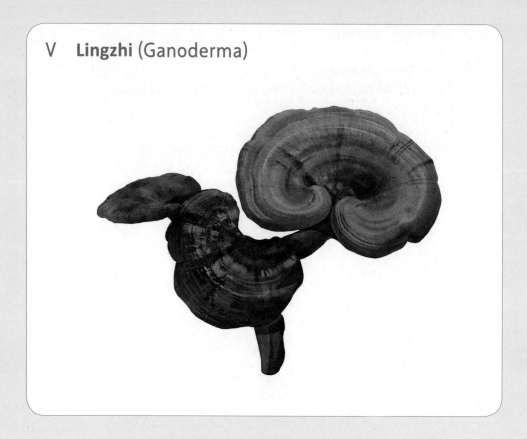

[Drug Selection by the Pharmacist]

◎ *How many kinds of Lingzhi (Ganoderma) are there? Which one is better?*

There are many species of Lingzhi (Ganoderma), including green, red, white, purple, and so on. It is generally believed that red and purple ones have great medicinal value.

◎ *How to distinguish the quality of Lingzhi (Ganoderma)?*

The choice of Lingzhi (Ganoderma) can be judged by its shape, color, thickness, and specific gravity. The fruiting body of Lingzhi (Ganoderma) with good quality has a short stalk, thick flesh. When the back or bottom of the fungus cap is observed with a magnifying glass, pores can be seen. The ones in light yellow or golden yellow color is best, followed by white and larges pores in gray white color are the worst.

◎ *How to preserve Lingzhi (Ganoderma)?*

Fresh Lingzhi (Ganoderma) can be eaten directly, but its storage life is very short. After fresh Lingzhi (Ganoderma) is collected, remove the silt and dust on the surface, dry naturally or by baking until the moisture is controlled below 13%, and then it is packed in a sealed bag and stored in a cool and dry place.

◎ *How to identify wild Lingzhi (Ganoderma)?*

Compared with cultivated Lingzhi (Ganoderma), wild Lingzhi (Ganoderma) is often more natural in color. Because of different species, it is usually different in size. Sometimes there are irregular worm holes under the fruiting body, and the taste is bitter.

**[Efficacy Told by the Doctor]**

◎ *Medicinal properties and efficacy—invigorating qi and nourishing blood, nourishing the heart and calming the mind, relieving cough and panting*

Lingzhi (Ganoderma) is sweet, slightly bitter, and not biased and enters the heart, lung, liver, and kidney meridians. TCM believes that sweet medicinals can tonify and moderate, so Lingzhi (Ganoderma) can tonify qi and blood; entering the heart meridian it can also nourish the heart and tranquillize the mind, and entering the lung meridian it can also relieve cough and panting.

◎ *Applicable people—people with physical weakness, deficiency of qi and blood, restlessness, cough, and wheezing*

Lingzhi (Ganoderma) is mainly suitable for people with physical weakness, and can tonify qi of the five internal organs and regulate human immunity, especially suitable for those who are usually tired and weak, have reduced appetite, or palpitations, insomnia, amnesia, neurasthenia, cough, asthma and short breath, and can also be used for daily healthcare of the general population.

Those with deficiency of qi and blood are often tired and weak, short of breath and unwilling to talk, have pale or sallow complexion, and reduced appetite.

Patients with mental uneasiness mainly present palpitations, forgetfulness, insomnia, neurasthenia, and so on.

Patients with cough and wheezing mainly have weak cough, panting, shortness of breath, spontaneous sweating, and susceptibility to wind and cold.

◎ *Applicable syndrome*

Lingzhi (Ganoderma) can improve human immunity. It can be used for hypertension, hyperlipidemia, coronary heart disease, leukopenia, chronic viral hepatitis.

◎ *What kinds of people are not suitable for Lingzhi (Ganoderma)?*

Lingzhi (Ganoderma) is a good medicinal for invigorating qi and blood and prolonging life, which can be eaten by the general population. People who are allergic to Lingzhi (Ganoderma) are not suitable to take it. In addition, patients of excess syndrome, or with tendency or have excessive internal heat, and those who are energetic are also forbidden to take it.

## [Diet Therapy Recommended by the Doctor]

◎ *Usage and dosage of Lingzhi (Ganoderma) in diet therapy*

Lingzhi (Ganoderma) is sweet and gentle, and 5–15g can be used as a substitute for tea in daily life. It can also be used to cook soup and congee and make Lingzhi (Ganoderma) wine.

◎ *What season is Lingzhi (Ganoderma) most suitable for taking?*

Lingzhi (Ganoderma) is mild and can be taken all year round.

◎ *How to combine Lingzhi (Ganoderma) with other medicinal materials and food ingredients?*

Lingzhi (Ganoderma) is often used with Huangqi (Astragali Radix) and

Danggui (Angelicae Sinensis Radix) to treat deficiency of qi and blood. Together with Dazao (Jujubae Fructus), Lianzixin (Nelumbinis Plumula) and Baihe (Lilii Bulbus), it is used for palpitation and insomnia. Combined with Renshen (Ginseng Radix et Rhizoma), Baihe (Lilii Bulbus) and Nanshashen (Adenophorae Radix), it is used for cough and asthma.

Lingzhi (Ganoderma) can be sliced alone to boil for drinking as tea, or it can be cooked as soup or congee with lean meat, Lianzi (Nelumbinis Semen), Baihe (Lilii Bulbus), etc., to clear the heart and tranquillize the mind. It can also be used to make Lingzhi (Ganoderma) wine, which is often used for neurasthenia, insomnia, indigestion, cough and asthma, senile bronchitis, and other diseases.

### Small experiential recipe

*1. To treat spleen deficiency and weak qi with reduced appetite, emaciation, and fatigue*

Lingzhi (Ganoderma) 30g and 1 chicken. Put Lingzhi (Ganoderma), ginger, pepper, salt, and wine into the chicken belly, add a proper amount of water, and steam until the chicken is thoroughly cooked. Eat the chicken and soup.

*2. To treat neurasthenia*

Lingzhi (Ganoderma) 6–9g, boil as tea and drink before going to bed.